160 YEARS OF SERVICE TO THE COMMUNITY

A HISTORY OF NEWMARKET GENERAL HOSPITAL

by Dick Heasman
Compiled and edited by John R Melleney

Published by Mid Anglia Community Health NHS Trust
Newmarket Hospital, Exning Road, Newmarket, Suffolk CB8 7JG

First published 1996

© Mid Anglia Community Health NHS Trust 1996

Typeset in 10pt Linotype Helvetica
by Focus 80 Ltd.,
Cowley Road, Cambridge CB4 4WX

ISBN 0 9528111 0 3

CONTENTS

Foreword		4
The Heasman Family		7
A Preface - Newmarket General Hospital		9
Chapter One	A Brief History of Hospitals in this Country	11
Chapter Two	Other Local Hospitals	21
Chapter Three	The Newmarket Union Workhouse	25
Chapter Four	The Infirmary Wards	35
Chapter Five	The Casual Wards	49
Chapter Six	The Public Assistance Institution	53
Chapter Seven	White Lodge Emergency Hospital - The War Years	59
Chapter Eight	The National Health Service - Secondary Care or Hospital Services	83
Chapter Nine	West Suffolk Hospital Management Committee	117
Chapter Ten	The First Reorganisation of the NHS	133
Chapter Eleven	The Restructured NHS 1982	145
Chapter Twelve	The Troubled Decade 1983 - 1993	149
Chapter Thirteen	The Church	167
Chapter Fourteen	The Redevelopment Saga	173
Chapter Fifteen	Tabulated History of Newmarket General Hospital	187
Index		198

FOREWORD

This history of Newmarket General Hospital is a labour of love on the part of Dick Heasman, whose family had direct links with the administration of the site for over sixty-six years.

Dick, who worked at the hospital site from 1932 until he retired on 13th July, 1977, clearly used the time between his retirement and death on 31st December, 1987, to do much of the work associated with writing the history. This must have involved, as will be seen from the text, a great deal of research into old minute books and registers as well as his own memory of events and people.

Why has this labour of love taken so long then to be published? In 1988, I was involved as Chief Executive of the then West Suffolk Health Authority, in presenting a manuscript and exhibition of items commemorating the fortieth anniversary of the National Health Service in West Suffolk. (It will be recalled that the NHS came about on 5th July, 1948.) My office was in touch with a large number of staff, former staff, patients and members of the public for mementoes of the period for the exhibition and we were able to contact Dick's brother, Reg, who himself had spent his working life in hospital administration. He indicated that Dick's manuscript of the history was in his possession and asked whether it was of interest to us. We obtained the documents which were typed but clearly incomplete since there were many penned alterations and additions made to it.

Writing such a history is something that retired people take to more easily than someone who is in full-time and demanding employment. It was not possible for me to pick up this happy task until I too retired and could find someone prepared to sponsor its publication. Happily, the Mid Anglia Community Health NHS Trust agreed to do so and it has now been reprocessed and published as the history.

Apart from this foreword, the pages on the Heasman family links with Newmarket and the caring services generally, the chapter on The Church and the final chapters relating to Newmarket after 1982, which clearly Dick could not have written, it is all his own work. I have presumed that amendment of his typing mistakes and of some grammatical and punctuation errors, which I have attempted to put right, would be acceptable. I have also taken the liberty of editing a little of his written material because although his views and opinions on matters of the day were his own, some of his references are best left unwritten. I have, however, deposited the <u>complete</u> text with his family and with the County Archives office in Bury St. Edmunds, for posterity and for reference by those who might wish to read his complete and unexpurgated version!

Whilst gritting my teeth on occasions on reading what he has written about events, knowing as I do from a similar length of service in the NHS as he, and from several different perspectives as a Hospital Secretary, Deputy House Governor, District Administrator and District General Manager, that his view was not necessarily one that would be shared within the whole profession, I have scrupulously avoided changing his words or editing out any text with which I did not agree. I repeat, it is all his own, loving work and one cannot fail to see his love of the local hospital, his high regard for staff and for the people of Newmarket in all he has written.

It would be too easy to write a history from reference to minutes books and reports, but without love of the subject and a very keen memory to recall the many anecdotal stories he has written, it would be dull reading. I believe, although there is a lot of text, he was successful in putting just enough detail to appeal to readers who have been patients, former members of the staff, or who have memories of the "good old days" passed down by parents or grandparents.

Apart from the additional chapters mentioned above, the only other addition I have made to the text is the inclusion of details of Acts of Parliament and other statutory documents, giving the full name and year where I could find it and the addition of a number of photographs and illustrations of Newmarket General Hospital in its existence since 1836.

I trust your reading of the history will also be a labour of love.

**J. R. Melleney.
January, 1996**

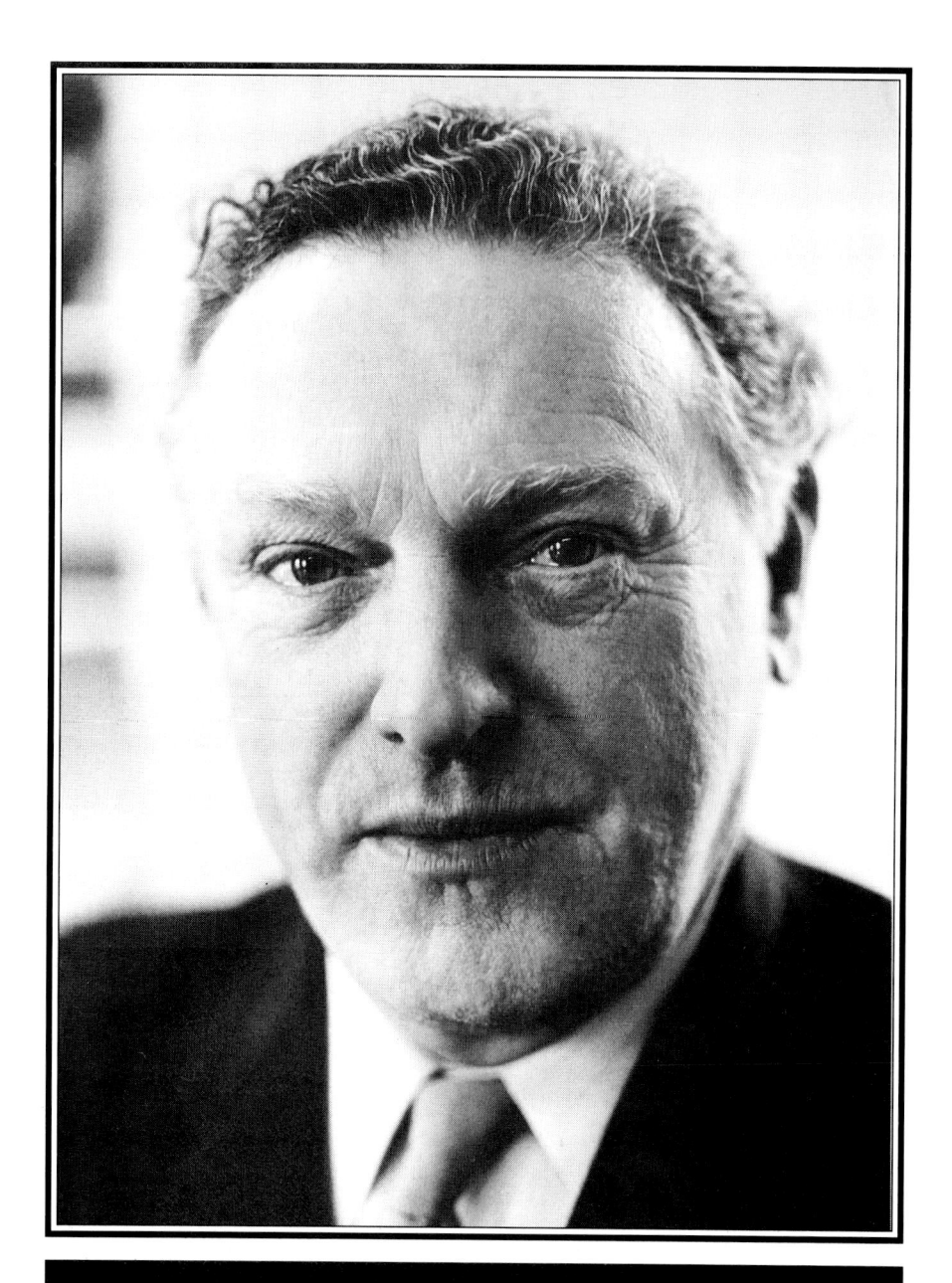

Richard Heasman

Photograph courtesy of Cambridge Evening News

THE HEASMAN FAMILY

Richard William Heasman (Dick), Fellow of the Institute of Health Service Administrators (FHA) died on 31st December, 1987, having retired some ten years earlier from his post of Hospital Secretary at Newmarket General Hospital, bringing to an end a Heasman family connection with Newmarket Hospital services of over sixty-six years. The family tree shows a unique and meritorious commitment to the health and caring services.

The maternal grandfather, William Livock, who died on 14th September, 1932, was Master of the Enfield Poor Law Institution (now St. Michael's Hospital, Enfield): his brother, Edward, was Superintendent of Chase Farm Poor Law Schools, which became Chase Farm Hospital, Enfield.

William's daughter, Ada Violet Livock, was born on 3rd May, 1887, qualified SRN, SCM, trained at St. Alphege's Hospital, now Greenwich District Hospital, from 1908 to 1911, and married Ernest Stephen Heasman on 19th March, 1912. Ernest, who was born on 25th September, 1884 and was also FHA, had a lifetime in public service, working as a junior clerk in the Sudbury Poor Law Institution (now Walnutree Hospital in Sudbury) from 1898, moving as Clerk to the Enfield Poor Law Institution from 1900 to 1905. He became Chief Clerk, Nottingham City Hospital from 1905 to 1907, Assistant Master of St. Marylebone Poor Law Institution from 1907 to 1911, Master of Newmarket Poor Law Institution from March 1911 until January 1942, when he was redesignated Clerk and Steward, Newmarket General Hospital, where he remained in post until March 1951. He died on 28th April 1970. His wife, Ada, was Matron with him from 1912 to 1942.

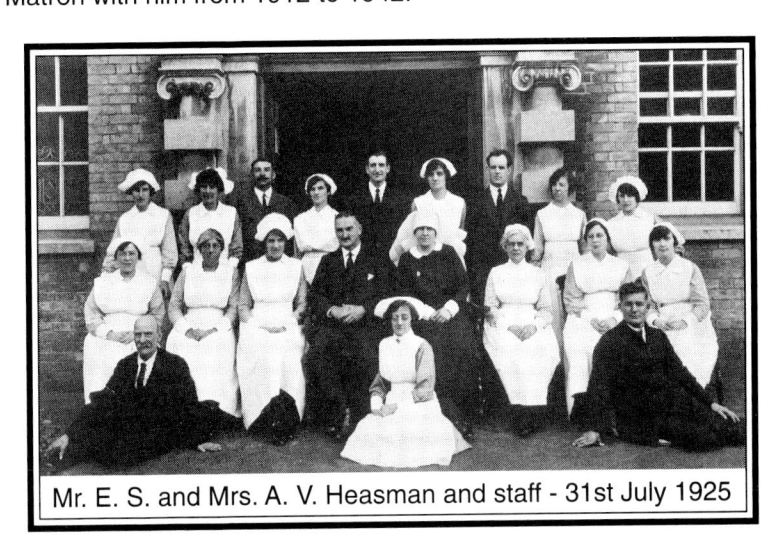

Mr. E. S. and Mrs. A. V. Heasman and staff - 31st July 1925

During their lifetime, Ada and Ernest Heasman produced two sons - George Reginald Livock (Reg) and Richard William (Dick), both of whom were to follow in their parents' career footsteps.

The first son, Reg, was born on 11th September, 1915 and was a junior clerk in the Newmarket Public Assistance Institution from 1932 to 1934 and moved through other Public Assistance Institutions in Epping, Lincoln, Watford, Leicester and York by 1949, having a break in service of some six years during the war years, where he served in the Field Artillery in the Middle East and Italy. He became Deputy Hospital Secretary, King Edward VII Hospital, Windsor, from 1949 to 1955, Hospital Secretary at Upton Hospital, Slough, from 1955 to 1960, Hospital Secretary at the Royal Devon and Exeter Hospital (Heavitree) from 1960 to 1975, and Sector Administrator, Exeter Acute Hospitals from 1975 to May 1980, when he retired, settling in Ebford, near Exeter.

Reg's wife, Rosanna Richardson, was born on 18th February, 1923, was also in the hospital service, qualifying SRN, SCM, RSCN. They married in March, 1951 and had two sons, both following health service careers. John Richard, born in 1953, after gaining an ONC in Business Studies, worked in hospital administrative posts in Exeter, Peterborough, Sidcup, Plymouth and as Hospital Secretary for Upton Hospital, Slough. He died in December, 1982. Michael Stephen, born in 1955, following his mother's career, qualified SRN in Starcross and is now a Charge Nurse for Exmouth Community Mental Handicap Services where he has been since 1980.

Dick, a lifelong bachelor, was born on 2nd May, 1917, and spent all of his working life in Newmarket. He became Junior Clerk at Newmarket Public Assistance Institution, working under his father, in 1934, was promoted to Senior Clerk in 1938 and from 1940 served with the Royal Corps of Signals as a Major, serving with the Chindits in Burma. He became Assistant Clerk and Steward, Newmarket General Hospital from 1946 to 1951, Assistant Hospital Secretary from 1951 to 1967 and Hospital Secretary from 1st April, 1967 working in this post until he retired on 13th July, 1977.

Dick was a keen cricketer with Exning Cricket Club and spent much of his leisure time at Southwold where he had a fishing boat. He alternated between living in Southwold and Newmarket during his ten years of retirement. He died on 31st December, 1987.

A PREFACE - NEWMARKET GENERAL HOSPITAL

The Hospital, like many others, started life as a Union of Parish Houses or Workhouses and has had a number of titles and played different roles since the first part of it was built nearly 160 years ago.

Built in 1836, as a central house to accommodate local able-bodied people who were destitute and had no work or anywhere to live, it was extended in 1890 to include an Infirmary to accommodate people who were sick and unable to work.

In 1930 it was upgraded and became a Public Assistance Institution under the administration of the West Suffolk County Council in Bury St. Edmunds. It was one of the main infirmaries working alongside Addenbrooke's Hospital in Cambridge, the main Voluntary Hospital in the area.

In 1939 and during the years of the second world war it was further upgraded and extensively extended to become one of the large Emergency Service Hospitals (E.M.S.) serving the vast number of Service personnel, stationed all over East Anglia and training for war. At the end of the war it was reported that over 30,000 mainly Service patients had been admitted to the hospital since 1939.

The years between the end of war in 1945 and the inception of the National Health Service in 1948 were difficult and a period of uncertainty for most hospitals. The White Lodge E.M.S. Hospital, as it was then known, was in a very bad state of repair and needed considerable upgrading and modification if is was to continue as a general hospital in civilian life. Money was very short and much of the limited equipment was coming to the end of its useful life. Staff who had been directed to work at the hospital during the war were returning to their homes and the poor pay structures made recruitment difficult. The military services and service patients were withdrawn or transferred to other hospitals and civilian patients were being admitted in their place.

The introduction of the National Health Service in l948 established the hospital as a General Hospital and provided a much better service all round. The South West No. 1 Group Hospital Management Committee (HMC) was founded, based at and worked as part of the General Hospital. The HMC was disbanded in May 1967, a few years before the first major reorganisation of the Health Service in April, 1974.

The unfortunate Cambridgeshire/Suffolk County boundary around Newmarket has affected the hospital and, at the time of writing, continues to do so. Since the war years the hospital has become orientated to Cambridgeshire with strong ties with Addenbrooke's Hospital in Cambridge. When the HMC was disbanded it was expected that the hospital would in future be administered by the Cambridge Hospitals Management Committee (the Board of Governors of the United Cambridge Hospitals) but it was put under the control of the West Suffolk HMC at Bury St. Edmunds. The psychiatric service was almost non-existent for the people residing in the Suffolk part of the town. Difficulties were also experienced with the Ambulance, Fire, Social Services, etc. For a long time the stretchers in the Cambridgeshire ambulances would not fit into the Suffolk ambulances.

Whatever the administrative changes the quality of work carried out in the hospital always depends on the skill and devotion of individual members of staff and it is the teamwork as a whole on which the reputation of a hospital is based. Newmarket General has always set a very high standard.

Staff recruitment has always been difficult. To an extent this is the result of a comparatively large hospital being located in a rather small town with its specialised horse racing industry.

The excellent support from the local people, both in the form of voluntary work and financial support, has played a very important part in the work of the hospital and the staff are always grateful for it. The Newmarket Journal Xmas Fund, the Hospital League of Friends, the local Lions Club and Mr. George Gibson are only a few who have helped consistently.

Only a few members of staff have been mentioned in this history. It is not possible to mention them all although they are worthy of it.

The wards and other accommodation have been put to many different uses and only some have been mentioned.

The wards and buildings, erected at the beginning of the war in 1939/40, were only intended to last for ten years and all the hospital buildings have been altered and modified so many times since it was started in 1836 to meet the varying needs of the service. They have now come to the end of their useful life and it is very good news to learn that in the autumn of 1982 the Department of Health agreed to build a new hospital on the existing site.

R. W. Heasman, 1987.

Chapter One

A BRIEF HISTORY OF HOSPITALS IN THIS COUNTRY

The first known hospitals were found in Turkey at Caesarea and Istanbul. The one in Caesarea was of immense size but, apart from this, very little else is known about them.

Broadly speaking, the history of the hospitals in Britain fall into seven main phases:

(1) Phase I 900 - 1500.

In Britain, as elsewhere throughout Christendom, the hierarchy of the Church and the Monastic rulers had accepted the obligation to provide hospitals for the sick and destitute. The history of our medieval hospitals extends over a period of some six and a half centuries until the suppression of the monasteries by Henry VIII.

The population of England was comparatively small and there was very little trade or movement of manpower. The Church was against learning which led to the stagnation of science and medicine. Disease was considered the penalty of sin and most of the progressive work for the sick was done by monks separate from the Church. The infirmarium or sick bay was an accepted part of the monastic institutions and merged almost imperceptibly into the "bedehouse" whose needy inmates were expected to pray for the souls of the founders. Such institutions must have been numerous from the days of the arrival of St. Augustin at Canterbury in 1596, since many traces of them still survive.

In France, the reign of Charlemagne (768-814) was marked by the foundation of hospitals of various kinds all over his Kingdom and the movement seems to have spread to England for a Saxon hospital is mentioned at St. Albans in 794 and was followed by others. St. Peters in York was founded in 937.

With the arrival of the Normans the establishment of hospitals accompanied the building of castles and cathedrals. Some eight hundred such foundations have been found.

During the 11th to 14th centuries the Church was still a barrier to the progress of medicine although it did encourage sympathy and help for the poor and suffering and became the main centre for "alms giving" and refuge for wayfarers.

Gradually the growth of industry resulted in an army of beggars and from 1388 onwards there was a form of legislation aimed at punishing the able-bodied who refused to work. These statutes were the forerunners of the Vagrancy Acts. There was still the problem of those people who were unable to work and those who could find none.

The dissolution of the monasteries by Henry VIII increased the difficulties of providing relief for the poor for it was originally regarded as a matter of private charity. The early legislation made use of charitable donations for this purpose. It is interesting to note that the parson, at the end of the Lesson, had to extort his parishioners to give liberally. Later the Bishop was made to take a hand if anyone refused to give his share. In the end the justices had to compel the obstinate man to cough up!

Finally, there was a provision that Church Wardens were to assess every man in the parish for his fair contribution. The unit of poor relief become the ecclesiastical unit of administration in the Parish.

The Poor Law legislation dates from the 1500's and was originally set up to ensure that each parish was responsible for providing relief for its own poor or paupers.

An Act of 1601 put upon the parish the burden of putting its unemployed able-bodied to work, or setting the children to work or putting them out as apprentices and of relieving the lame, impotent, old, blind and other persons who were not able to work. The actual duties were imposed on the Church Wardens and certain new officials, the overseers, appointed by the Justices of each Parish. The cost was to be met by the occupiers of property in the Parish. This seems to be where our system of domestic rates started!

Over the ensuing years a vast but very inefficient system of social welfare relief for the poor grew up, subject to changes in government policy, public opinion and local interpretation. During the 1700's a fairly humane interpretation was placed on the laws.

(2) Phase II 1500 - 1750

In the year 1534 Henry VIII broke with the Pope. The Court and the great merchant community of the towns and countryside became aggressively Protestant. Thomas Cromwell embarked on his famous series of Statutes (1536-1547) for the suppression of religious houses. It was not possible for the hospitals, such as they were, to be exempt for they were first and foremost religious houses. The great majority of hospitals were surrendered.

Soon the lack of hospitals became intolerable and this led to the creation of the Royal Hospitals, really civic hospitals, in London and after about 200 years, in the 18th century, the building of the Voluntary Hospitals. With the formation of the Royal Hospitals in London a new spirit of open minded enquiry into medicine was seen and in all the Universities of Europe questions were being asked and scientific surgery was being born.

The Voluntary Hospitals were essentially a partnership between doctors and enterprising laymen willing to provide for the needs of the sick so far as their means permitted.

The Voluntary Hospital system spread and went far and wide throughout the cities and larger towns of the Kingdom, creating hospitals which became household names. 31 Voluntary hospitals were built in Britain in the 18th century and by 1825 no less than 124 hospitals and dispensaries had been established.

A number of these hospitals which, geographically, would be of interest are:

> Northampton General Hospital   built 1743.
> Addenbrooke's Hospital, Cambridge   built 1766.
> Norfolk & Norwich Hospital   built 1772.

(3) Phase III 1750 - 1939.

In 1782 an Act of Parliament was passed, known as the Gilbert Act, giving parishes powers to unite to form an incorporative and build houses for the sick and aged. The able-bodied were to be found suitable labour near their homes.

Early in the 1800's public opinion swung against providing relief for the poor persons. One result of this was the Poor Law Commission in 1832 and an amendment Act in 1834. This led to the grouping of parishes by a Board of Guardians for the government of workhouses and the classification of inmates. The Act also reflected the feeling that pauperism had some moral stigma and that the aim should now be to discourage people from becoming paupers, rather than relieving their position when they were in that state. As a result the aim was to make the instruments of poor relief, such as workhouses, very austere and by making these conditions so unpleasant, discourage people from ever reaching the state where they might have to make use of them.

Gradually Poor Law took on a much larger connotation and tended to attract to itself many other functions. The Guardians began to provide Infirmaries and other medical relief for the sick, orphans, education of children, special accommodation for lunatics and mental defectives and the blind. The union and workhouse system was introduced throughout the country about this time.

An Act of 1867 made provision for Poor Law Infirmaries separate from Workhouses but only comparatively few of these were built. This arrangement continued until responsibilities were transferred to Local Authorities in 1929. From 1930 until the National Health Service was introduced in 1948 some workhouses and infirmaries became the Public Health hospitals working alongside the Voluntary hospitals.

The high hopes of the new era brought about by the transfer of responsibilities to Local Authorities were only partly realised. The more prosperous areas made great strides in bringing the old Infirmaries up to a standard compared to that of the better Voluntary Hospitals but, unfortunately, other poorer areas lagged behind and despite the equalising effect of subsidies from the Exchequer, were unable to meet the expense of modernising old hospitals or building new ones. It was already apparent before the war that the time had come for a fresh attempt to weld together the Voluntary and Local Authority Public hospitals into a single system. This was envisaged in a report by Lord Dawson as early as 1920.

(4) Phase IV 1940 - 1948

When war came the prospects of casualties on a great scale meant that a national service had to be improvised, sufficiently elastic to admit the transference of cases from one hospital to another and in the last few months before the start of war hospitals were grouped together in the Emergency Hospital Service. Doctors, Nurses, Matrons and Administrators were drawn from different units and given a quasi-military status in their respective areas.

When the first casualties arrived from Dunkirk in 1940 and, later throughout the war years, the system worked smoothly and it was realised that many elements of the improvisations ought to be embodied into a permanent structure.

Hospital accommodation for military patients was made available in the following types of hospitals:

a. Military Hospitals.
b. Civil Hospitals of the Emergency Medical Service of the Ministry of Health. Newmarket Hospital was one of these.
c. Ministry of Pension Hospitals.
d. Certain Civil Hospitals not included in the EMS, e.g. Infectious Diseases Hospitals.
e. Convalescent Hospitals run by the British Red Cross Society and Order of St. John of Jerusalem.

Arrangements were made for the treatment of special types of cases at special hospitals, e.g. 18 EMS Hospitals specialised in orthopaedic cases, 9 specialised in facial injury, 9 in head injuries, 9 in chest wounds, 8 in cases of neurosis and 18 in diseases of the skin.

The precise condition of each patient was stipulated to ensure only suitable cases were sent to those centres.

London was divided into ten Administration Sectors and outside London twelve Administration Regional Centres were formed.

By 1944 the EMS had developed considerably and the hospitals were admitting patients in twenty-six different classifications: these included civilians, prisoners of war, Service and ex-Service cases, evacuated children, refugees from abroad and so on. Many had to be charged for their treatment and services. Standard systems for statistics, medical records and costings were set up. It was a shame that the revised national systems were not retained in the National Health Service introduced in 1948.

Although there were quite a number of private and other types of hospitals which remained outside the EMS Service, there is no doubt it was the basis of the new National Health Service introduced in 1948.

(5) Phase V 1948 - 1974

It was now clear that a single authority of health service administration was necessary if a balanced pattern of care in the homes (primary care) or in hospitals (secondary care) was to be developed.

The initial proposals of the British Coalition Government in the early 1940's for the creation of the National Health Service, showed a similar belief in the desirability of unified health service direction but, unfortunately, some of the influential groups in health care at the time, notably the British Medical Association, feared that their position and the interests of their members would be undermined if such a structure was adopted. Hence a compromise was adopted when the N.H.S. was formed on 5th July, 1948. This involved the administrative separation of the local authority services, hospitals, consultant medical staff and general practitioners, who became independent contractors to the Service. The Local Authorities remained responsible for the primary health care, i.e. school health services, district nurses, the ambulance service and local health clinics.

A new system of administration was introduced for the secondary care in hospitals. Fourteen Regional Hospital Boards (RHB) were set up throughout the country to administer small groups of hospitals, through Hospital Management Committees (HMC). The thirty-six Boards of Governors of Teaching Hospitals remained. Most hospitals had its own House Committee for the day to day work and the HMC group headquarters was usually based on the main hospital in the group. In this area it is interesting to note the S.W. No. 1 Group Hospital Management Committee was based at Newmarket General Hospital.

The aim of the NHS was to make all heath services available to every man, woman and child in the population and to make the total cost of the service a charge on the National Income.

The framework of the original NHS in 1948 was:

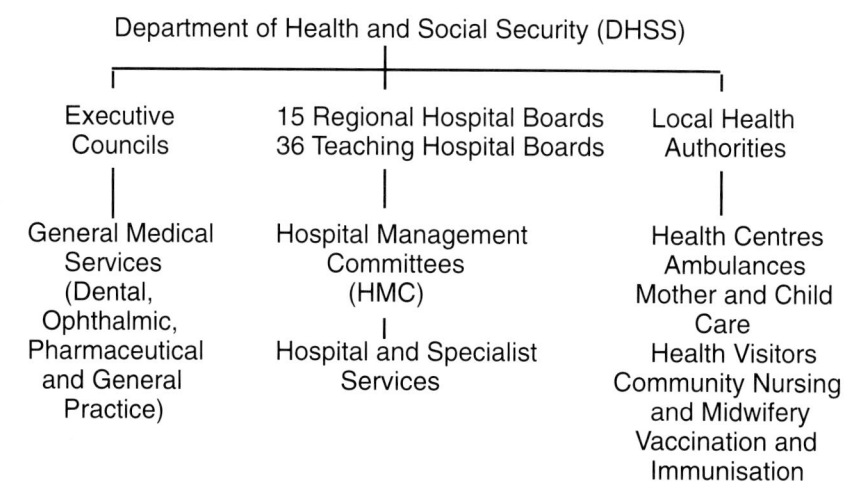

Department of Health and Social Security (DHSS)

Executive Councils	15 Regional Hospital Boards 36 Teaching Hospital Boards	Local Health Authorities
General Medical Services (Dental, Ophthalmic, Pharmaceutical and General Practice)	Hospital Management Committees (HMC) Hospital and Specialist Services	Health Centres Ambulances Mother and Child Care Health Visitors Community Nursing and Midwifery Vaccination and Immunisation

(6) Phase VI 1974 - 1981

The NHS system was in the short term a workable answer to the many problems encountered in the past. It was certainly an improvement and its progress was watched closely by other countries all over the world. During the first twenty-five years of its existence deficiencies were clearly revealed.

The compromise of leaving a large section of primary care outside of the hospital service was troublesome and in the 1960's pressure began to grow, notably with the publication of the Porritt report in 1962, for a more uniform service. In 1968 the Labour Government expressed its intention to act towards a single tier system of administration.

A great deal of authority had been given to the numerous HMC up and down the country and with an ever increasing flow of instructions coming direct from the DHSS, the RHB had very little administrative control over them. Standards and systems differed and instead of a uniform service a system more like a patchwork quilt existed.

The date imposed on the first reorganisation was 1st April, 1974, which coincided with the reorganisation of Local Government.

The changes in management introduced in the reorganised health service structure owe their origin to a number of sources. These include a firm of American Management Consultants, McKinsey, and the work of the Brunel Health Service Organisation Unit. Political considerations and pressures applied by representative groups, such as the British Medical Association, also played an important part in determining many aspects of the reorganisation. There was a strong feeling in the Service at that time that the Management Consultants, McKinsey, should never have been appointed for this work. They had no experience of a National Health Service and sometime later when they reviewed their recommendations they admitted publicly that there were major defects in its present form.

The services brought together under the reorganised Service were:

a. the Hospital Service.
b. Ambulance Service.
c. Family Planning.
d. Health Centres.
e. Health Visiting.
f. Home Nursing and Midwifery.
g. Vaccination and immunisation.
h. the School Health Service.
i. the dental, ophthalmic, pharmaceutical and family doctor service.

The services still remaining outside of the Health Service included:

a. the occupational health service of the Department of Employment.

b. the environmental health service, run by Local Authorities with NHS consultant advice.

c. the personal social services including hospital social work previously carried out by the Hospital Almoners.

d. certain other health provisions, e.g. prison health service and services for the armed forces.

The overall framework of the 1974 reorganised NHS looked like this:

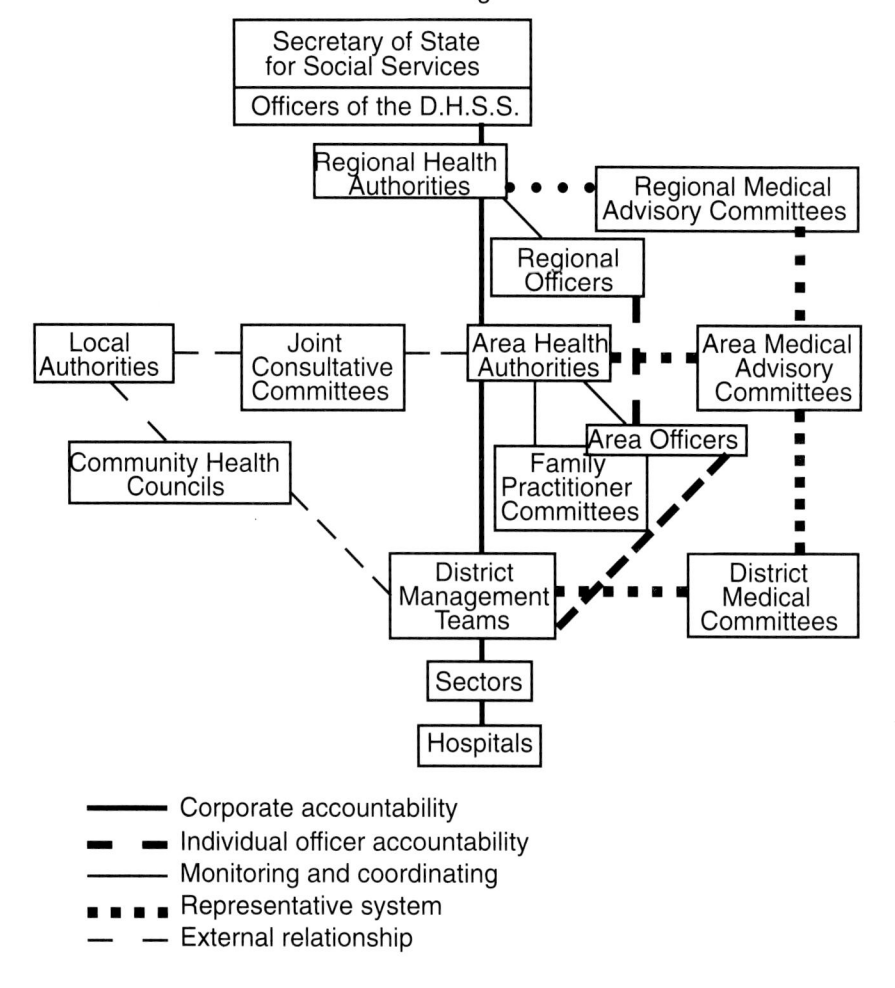

```
        ┌─────────────────────────┐
        │ Secretary of State      │
        │ for Social Services     │
        ├─────────────────────────┤
        │ Officers of the D.H.S.S.│
        └─────────────────────────┘
                    │
        ┌─────────────────────┐         ┌─────────────────────┐
        │ Regional Health     │ • • • • │ Regional Medical    │
        │ Authorities         │         │ Advisory Committees │
        └─────────────────────┘         └─────────────────────┘
                    │       ┌──────────────┐
                    │       │ Regional     │
                    │       │ Officers     │
                    │       └──────────────┘
┌──────────┐  ┌──────────────┐  ┌──────────────┐  ┌──────────────┐
│ Local    │──│ Joint        │──│ Area Health  │• │ Area Medical │
│Authorities│  │ Consultative │  │ Authorities  │• │ Advisory     │
│          │  │ Committees   │  │              │• │ Committees   │
└──────────┘  └──────────────┘  └──────────────┘  └──────────────┘
      \                                │ ┌──────────────┐
       \                               │ │ Area Officers│
   ┌─────────────────┐                 │ └──────────────┘
   │ Community Health│            ┌──────────────┐
   │ Councils        │            │ Family       │
   └─────────────────┘            │ Practitioner │
            \                     │ Committees   │
             \                    └──────────────┘
              \              ┌──────────────┐   ┌──────────────┐
               \             │ District     │   │ District     │
                \────────────│ Management   │•••│ Medical      │
                             │ Teams        │   │ Committees   │
                             └──────────────┘   └──────────────┘
                                    │
                             ┌──────────┐
                             │ Sectors  │
                             └──────────┘
                                    │
                             ┌──────────┐
                             │ Hospitals│
                             └──────────┘
```

────────── Corporate accountability
■ ■ ■ Individual officer accountability
────────── Monitoring and coordinating
■ ■ ■ ■ Representative system
— — External relationship

In England ninety Area Health Authorities (AHA) were added to the existing administrative structure. These had statutory responsibilities for running the health services at local level. It was not the slimmed down service hoped for.

The Grey Book, as it was known, ("Management Arrangements for the Reorganised National Health Service" published by H.M.S.O. in 1972) was the document which introduced the reorganised management system. It started in great detail at the top of the tree and worked downwards to district level. Only a brief mention was made of how the new system would work at the Sector level and in the Units of hospitals and in primary care. This was unfortunate since these are the levels containing the patients. I feel if they had started to reorganise at the patients' end and worked backwards quite a different management structure would have resulted. The confusion and duplication of decision making at all levels made life very difficult for the staff directly connected with the patients' care.

(7) Phase VII 1982

In 1982 the National Health Service was again restructured. Roughly speaking the extra tier of management - the Area introduced in the first reorganisation of 1974 - was removed. In place of the AHA, 192 Health Districts were created and to some extent individual hospitals came back into greater prominence administratively. The hospital departments also came under scrutiny and in some cases the structure and staffing altered. The dust had scarcely settled, an unfortunate expression perhaps in the circumstances, when it was abruptly restirred by the publication of the Griffiths report. This was the result of a NHS Management Inquiry resulting from a general opinion that the Health Service could be very much better managed than it was. The report recommended the appointment of General Managers at each level of the service, not necessarily hospital administrators but people with management experience who would run the services efficiently and make sure action on any issue could be taken quickly and effectively. It placed considerable authority in the hands of people holding these positions.

The rapid growth of private medicine and private hospitals and the way they were managed makes one wonder where this second reorganisation is going.

Unlike England, where the Area layer of management has been removed, in Scotland, roughly speaking, they have removed the District layer of management. It will be interesting to see, in time, just how the two different systems compare.

The vast number of reports, instructions, surveys, work studies, consultant's reports, etc. on the NHS would almost fill the Albert Hall. Very few are fully implemented and seem to have very little to do with the patients.

Chapter Two

OTHER LOCAL HOSPITALS

Although this is the history of Newmarket General Hospital it would be wrong not to mention other local hospitals whose work was involved and appreciated. They gave excellent service to the people of Newmarket and District.

The Rous Memorial Hospital was originally built in 1879 in memory of Admiral Rous, a great patron of the Turf, and on land given by Sir Richard Wallace. The general plan was for a pavilion, having beds for ten people. Patients were mainly admitted from the racing fraternity, although on occasions others were given treatment in emergency. In 1887 H.R.H. the Prince of Wales opened an extension to the hospital so that female patients could be admitted. The extension was a gift made by the inhabitants of Newmarket in celebration of Queen Victoria's Jubilee. Over time this little hospital was kept up to date and was really a small private General Hospital with connections with Addenbrooke's Hospital in Cambridge. Although its main purpose was to provide a service for the people in the horse racing industry it did very good work for the other sections of the population.

I am sure that many local people will remember this excellent little hospital which remained in being until the main Newmarket General Hospital was well established. It was purchased by the local Council in 1966 and converted into homes for the elderly people of Newmarket.

The Exning Isolation Hospital

Originally known as the town Fever Hospital it provided accommodation for patients suffering from infectious diseases such as smallpox, scarlet fever, etc. The spread of infection was a real danger, both in the home and in the hospitals, and patients were sent to the Isolation Hospital until the risk of infection had ceased. This small unit gave excellent service until the progress of medicine diminished its need. Its very location made it difficult to staff and although it was used as a geriatric unit for a short time it was finally closed at the end of August 1963. Many people in Exning will remember Mr. Varley who, as porter, gardener and jack of all trades, dedicated his life's work to this hospital. In 1962, in addition to his meagre wage, he was paid £4.00 per annum bicycle allowance.

Workhouses

About 1790, in line with the Gilbert Act, houses were built in the parishes of All

Saints and St. Mary's for the sick and aged. They were originally governed by the Overseers of the Parishes. A house in Parish Street and another near the Red House in St. Mary's Square are believed to have been built for this purpose. No doubt other parishes have knowledge of such houses in their area. In about 1830 a local Board of Guardians was formed to govern the union of these houses in the Newmarket area. They held their meetings in Kingston House rooms, Newmarket.

Fulbourn Asylum

Built very early on to accommodate mental cases, Fulbourn Asylum was located in Cambridgeshire and would only accept cases living in that county. In those early days the Cambridgeshire/Suffolk boundary ran down the centre of the high street of Newmarket and divided the town. The effect was that patients living in the All Saints (Cambridgeshire) side could be sent to Fulbourn, which was close by, whilst those living in the St. Mary's and Exning side (Suffolk) had to be sent all the way to Melton Asylum, near Ipswich. This is only one difficulty thrown up by the silly County boundary which still exists.

Mildenhall Workhouse

The workhouse at Mildenhall was comparatively small and must have been in existence early in 1800 and undoubtedly records of this are in existence at Mildenhall. It was closed some years after, when the new workhouse at Newmarket was built. Much of the original equipment was transferred there. I remember as late as 1947 a number of large meat dishes marked in a circle "Mildenhall Workhouse" standing on a large old-fashioned wooden dresser in the original kitchen at Newmarket. I wonder whatever happened to them and what they would be worth today?

Cardigan Street District Nursing Home

The Cardigan Street District Nursing Home was built in 1923 by the Charities Commission in memory of the men who fought in the 1914-1918 war. In the autumn of 1954 the Commission kindly let the Hospital use the property as a maternity unit to relieve heavy bookings in the main unit. It was returned to the owners on 27th January, 1956.

United States Military Hospital - Lakenheath

This small general hospital was opened in May 1965 for the American Services personnel at the Lakenheath base. It enjoyed very good relationships with Newmarket General Hospital. Initially, for some reason, it had no main incinerators or sterilizers and the work was done at the Newmarket Hospital until their own equipment was available some two years later.

Chapter Three

THE NEWMARKET UNION WORKHOUSE

About 1830 the Guardians of the Newmarket Union of the Parish houses, who were also responsible for the administration of poor relief, had decided that there was a need for a new central workhouse in Newmarket. They commenced their meetings on 31st December, 1835, in the Kingston House rooms in Newmarket. At their meeting on 27th May, 1836, they recommended the purchase of 4 acres of land at a cost not exceeding £400 and for a workhouse to be built on the land at a sum not exceeding £7,500. On 12th July, 1836, the Poor Law Commissioners acknowledged receipt of a letter from the Guardians asking for an advance of £7,900 to carry out this work. Approval for the loan was given, which was just as well, because the work had already commenced in June 1836!

The main contractors were Messrs. Steggles of Newmarket and on 28th October they asked for an extension in time to complete the workhouse. The extension was until 24th December but, on 3rd February, 1837, the Clerk to Guardians of the Union was asked to write to the contractors, yet again, complaining about the delay in completing the building. The building was finished soon afterwards and the first meeting of the Board of Guardians was held on Saturday, 25th March, 1837, in the new Newmarket Workhouse Board Room.

When built the workhouse was located in a most isolated spot, well outside of the town. From Bakers Row to the workhouse there were no houses at all on either side of the Exning Road. The fields were separated from Exning Road by wooden fences. The Gas works and Electricity works had not been built and for about thirty-eight years the workhouse was the only building between Newmarket and Exning: the first houses were those in Gwynne Terrace in 1875. These adjoin the hospital premises and one of them had been used as a Fish and Chip shop for as long as I can remember. The inscriptions on other houses give a good indication when Field Terrace, St. Phillips and King Edward Roads came into being:

St. Phillip's Terrace	1898
Prospect Terrace	1891
Stamford Terrace	1882
Cherry Cottages	1882
Victoria Villa	1897
Norfolk Cottage - Field Terrace Road	1901
Foulden Terrace, the present Post Office	1902
Essex House	1913

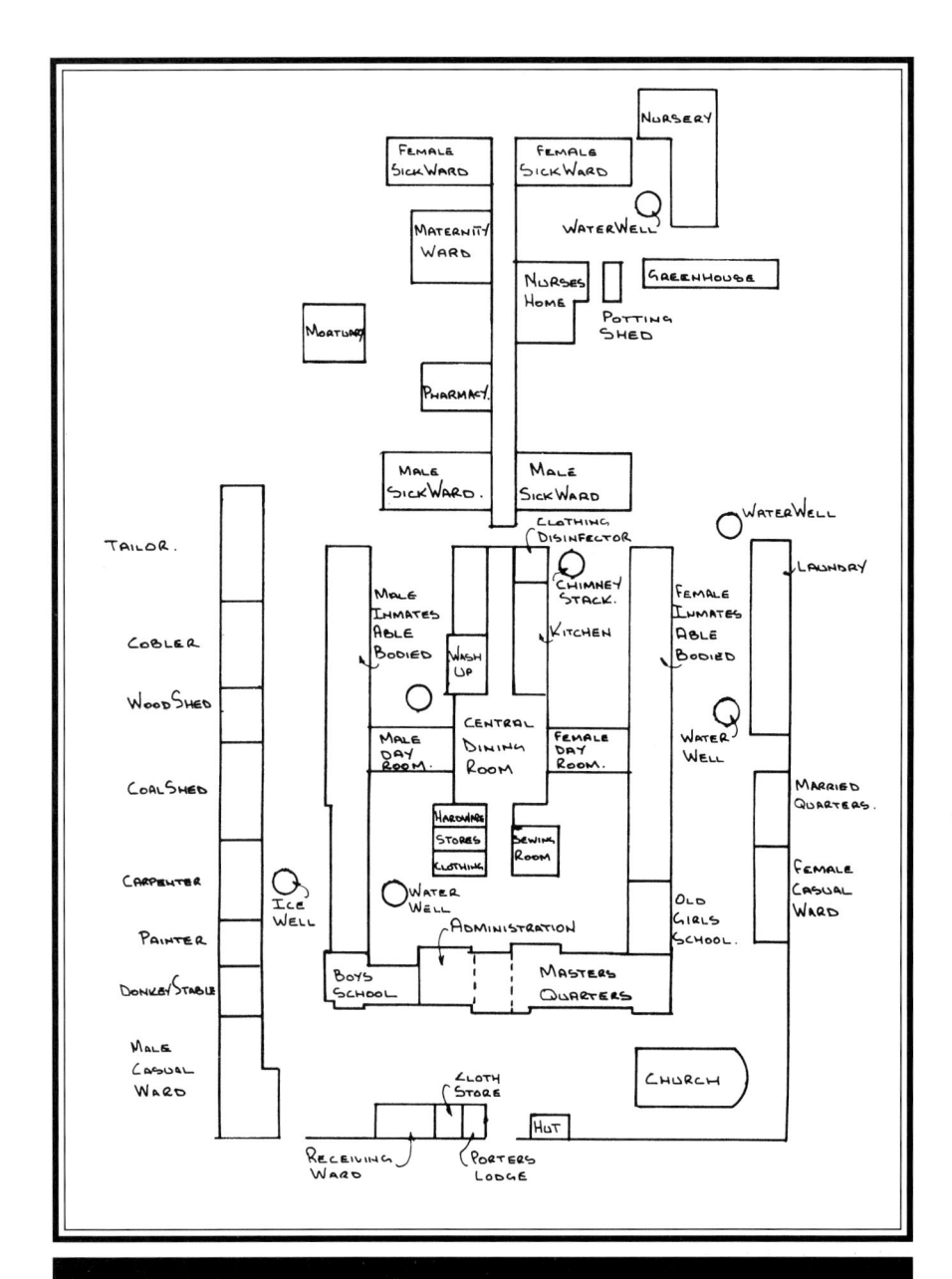

**Plan of
The Newmarket Union Workhouse 1836**

Essex House was the original Post Office run by the Wheeler family until after the second world war.

The majority of the workhouse accommodation was used for the able-bodied poor, since the main intention of the Poor Law was to look after these persons. It also provided short stay accommodation for tramps or casuals passing through the town.

About this time other Unions were built in the district at Bury St. Edmunds, Haverhill, Cambridge, Sudbury and Linton.

Separate accommodation was provided for males and females and there were a few cottages for married couples over 65 years old.

Separate boys' and girls' schoolrooms and stables for horses were also included, together with an infants' nursery for orphans, unwanted children and those children of mothers who needed help. A block diagram of the layout of the original workhouse is shown opposite.

In the 1800's public opinion swung against providing relief for the poor persons and the Poor Law Commission of 1832 and a new Poor Law Amendment Act of 1834, made administration more efficient and also reflected the feeling that pauperism had some moral stigma and the aim should now be to discourage people from becoming paupers, rather than relieving their position when they were in that state. The result was to make the instruments of poor relief, such as workhouses, very austere and by making conditions so unpleasant discourage people from ever reaching the state where they might have to make use of them.

Bearing in mind that inmates of the workhouse were poor, but able-bodied, people and the Newmarket Workhouse opened in the years of austerity that followed the 1834 Act, it is not surprising that the inmates were made to work to make the Institutions as self-supporting as possible.

The feeding arrangements are interesting. In a letter dated 30th April, 1836, the Poor Law Commission gave the following guidance:

> *"in making this selection (of diet) especial reference must be had to the usual mode of living of the Independent Labourers in the District in which the Union is situated and on no account must the Dietary of the Workhouse be superior or equal to the ordinary mode of subsistence of the labouring classes of the*

neighbourhood. Want of attention to this essential point has been the cause of much evil by too frequently exhibiting the Pauper Inmates of a Workhouse as fed, lodged and clothed in a way superior to Individuals subsisting by their own honest industry, thereby lessening the stimulus to exertion and holding out on inducement to idle and improvident habits."

If only we could apply something like this to the House of Commons today!!

The Poor Law Commission made a number of diets available: the choice was left to the Workhouse Committee. The following is an example:

BREAKFAST

		Bread	Gruel		
Sunday	Male	6 ozs.	1½ pints		
	Female	5 ozs.	1½ pints		

DINNER

		Cooked Meat	Potatoes	Soup	Suet/Rice Pudding
Sunday	Male	5 ozs.	½ lb		
	Female	5 ozs.	½ lb		
Monday	Male				1½ pints
	Female				1½ pints

SUPPER

		Bread	Cheese	Broth
Sunday	Male	6 ozs		1½ pints
	Female	5 ozs.		1½ pints
Monday	Male	6 ozs.	2 ozs.	
	Female	5 ozs.	2 ozs.	

A number of variations could be made for inmates who were over the age of 60. One letter stated "1 oz. tea, soup, butter, 7 ozs sugar per week in lieu of gruel for breakfast can be made available if deemed expedient to make this change."

Feeding for the sick, however, was totally at the discretion of the Medical Officer. They (the sick) could be provided with alcohol. In December 1839 the following quotation was received by the Workhouse Committee for the provision of spirits on the understanding that all the bottles were returnable:

Sherry	3/6 per bottle	Port	4/- per bottle
Brandy	31/- per gallon	Gin	11/- per gallon.

The Workhouse Committee tried to ameliorate these conditions and on 9th May, 1837, recorded the following minute:

"The Workhouse Committee ordered a certain quantity of beef and peas to be boiled with the paupers' soup with the purpose of rendering it more nutritional".

The Clerk was directed to write to the Poor Law Commissions for their sanction to make the above alteration in the diet.

It is not always easy to gain an accurate picture from the formal minute books but a number of items do help to give a picture of what life was like in the early years of this particular workhouse and also show what level of care was instituted by the Board of Guardians of the Newmarket Union.

An entry on 17th November, 1840, shows that the Board of Guardians had taken note of the recent medical advice on vaccination against smallpox and it was agreed at that meeting to draw up a legal contract with a qualified medical practitioner to ensure *"the vaccination of all persons resident in the Union"* and *"to do and perform all such Acts and things as may be necessary for the immediate purpose of causing such vaccination to be successfully terminated."*

The fee for each successful vaccination was 1/6d. to be paid to the medical practitioner and, in addition, the doctor was required to keep a register of all smallpox cases attended.

The legal terminology used in drawing up this contract should not disguise the fact that vaccination for smallpox was an important medical advance and it is interesting to note that this was made available to the poorest people in the community.

The medical officer had another important role to play in seeing that the conditions in the Workhouse did not reach a state whereby the inmates' health was affected. On 14th December, 1841, one wrote a letter to the Board of Guardians

"Sir, during my visit to the Workhouse this day, my attention was directed to the crowded state of the Apartments, especially to those on the women's side; these compartments contain already too many beds and each bed is made to contain too many inmates. (Medical Officer's underlining).

> *I should be wanting in my duty were I not to notice these facts respectfully for the consideration of the Guardians, urging the proprietary of thinning the apartments so as to secure the health of the Inmates, which I believe to be endangered by being too thickly packed."*

The Workhouse Committee noted that:

> *"the cleanliness of the bedrooms and ventilation of the house is not properly attended to"*

and moves were taken to reduce the number of inmates. In addition, the Governor was reprimanded for the dirty state of the Workhouse.

In January, 1842 there was further recorded:

> *"the Workhouse Committee reported that the single mens' ward was in a dirty state and much crowded and without proper control or discipline and the Mill was inefficient. Ordered that the Clerk advertise for an efficient person to superintend the working of the Mill."*

It was subsequently noted that two new millstones were ordered.

Perhaps as a result of these unhygienic conditions, the behaviour of some of the inmates left much to be desired:

> *"24th August, 1841 - Charlotte Beningfield, a pauper applying for relief, having conducted herself with great violence in the boardroom by dashing the chairs on the floor and otherwise misbehaving herself, was ordered to be given in charge to a Constable."*

and

> *"12th October, 1841 - the Master of the Workhouse reported that Christopher Shave, a pauper, had absconded from the Workhouse, leaving his wife and family."*

Finally, Dr. Platts kindly lent me a book "Fenwomen" by Mary Chamberlain, which contains a reminiscence that reflects on the life in the Workhouse in the 19th century. This reminiscence is by Gladys Otterspoor who, at the time the book was written, was 83 years old:

> "And families years ago, they used to pack up and go in the Workhouse for the winter. The women used to have to wash and the men had to do outside, round the garden. To earn their keep. And that's all they had all day. A bit of washing with a little skilly. That's all they were given. That's what my mother told me she'd been in. Hard times they wouldn't earn enough outdoor relief so they'd take the families into the Workhouse. You'd have to go for the winter couldn't do nothing at all, couldn't have a fire, couldn't do nothing. My mother say she packed up many a winter when she were a girl and been in the Workhouse. I used to say "no you ain't mother." She say "Yes, I have.""

The following extracts are taken from the Minute Books of 1851 and 1852 and show the wide variety of detailed interest that was taken by the Board of Guardians running both the Workhouse and the Poor Relief in the surrounding districts.

The minutes of a meeting on Friday, 2nd April, 1852, show that the powers of the Master were severely limited:

> "It was resolved that the Master be allowed a discretionary power of ordering repairs in and about the Workhouse in any cases of emergency but that he be required to report the same to the House Committee at the next ensuing Board Day."

The same set of minutes also shows continued interest in the medical care of the poor and the following was passed:

> "That the medical officers of this Union shall in future be paid by annual salary instead of the "per case" system (except in cases of fractures, operations, midwifery and vaccination)."

A separate sub-committee was then set up to consider the salaries of medical officers and "the mode of determining the proper objects for medical relief".

The most revealing section on the conditions within the Workhouse, however, comes in the minutes of a meeting of 20th February, 1852:

"A letter was read from the Poor Law Board stating that they had received a communication informing them that in order to provide employment for the Inmates of the Workhouse of this Union, white and black oats were intermixed; that the paupers were then required to separate the white from the black and that they were afterwards intermixed as before; also that children as early as one year and a half old were separated from their mothers all day."

The response to this novel form of work creation by the Poor Law Board showed the attempts by the Board of Guardians to soften some of these conditions:

"The Clerk was instructed to state to the Poor Law Board that the employment of separating white oats from black as described by them, had been introduced into the House, but that at the present time they had a supply of barley containing a mixture of seeds which the paupers were employed in separating for the purpose of putting the barley for use and consequently the different grains were not intermixed after being separated.

Also that the children remain constantly with their mothers until they are two years old."

The following poem was written in 1846 by J.R. Withers, Poet of Fordham, to his sister in Cambridge, from Union:

*"Since I cannot, dear sister, with you hold communion
I'll give you a sketch of our life in the Union.
But how to begin, I don't know, I declare
Let me see: well, the first is our grand bill of fare.
We've skilly for breakfast, at night bread and cheese
And we eat it and then go to bed if we please.
Two days in the week we've pudding for dinner
And two we have broth, so like water, but thinner.
Two meat and potatoes, of this none to spare;
One day bread and cheese and this is our fare.*

*And now then, my clothes, I will try to portray;
They're made, of coarse cloth and the colour is grey.
My jacket and waistcoat don't fit me at all,*

*My shirt is too short, or else I am too tall;
My shoes are not pairs, though of course I have two
They are down at the heel and my stockings are blue.

But what shall I say of the things they call breeches,
Why mine are so large they'd have fitted John Fitches,
John Fitches, you say, well pray who was he?
Why one of the fattest men I ever did see.
Neither breeches, nor trousers, but something between,
And though they're so large, you'll remember I beg,
That they're low on the waist and high on the leg.

And no braces allowed me oh dear, oh dear!
We are each other's glass, so I know I look queer,
A sort of Scotch bonnet we wear on our heads,
And I sleep in a room where there are just fourteen beds.
Some are sleeping, some swearing, but very few praying.

Here are nine at a time who work on the mill,
We take it by turns, so it never stands still,
A half an hour each gang, 'tis not very hard
And when we are off we can walk in the yard.
We have nurseries here, where the children are crying,
And hospitals, too, for the sick and the dying.

But I must not forget to record in my verse,
All who die here are honoured to ride in a hearse.
I sometimes look up at a bit of blue sky
High over my head, with a tear in my eye,
Surrounded by walls that are too high to climb,
Confined as a felon without any crime.
Not a field, not a house, not a hedge can I see,
Not a plant, not a flower, not a bush, nor a tree,
Except a geranium or two appear
At the Governor's window, to smile, even here.

But I find I am got too pathetic by half,
And my object was only to cause you a laugh,
So my lover to yourself, your husband and daughter,
I'll drink to your health in a tin of cold water.
Of course, we've no wine, nor porter, nor beer,
So you see that we are all teetotallers here."*

# Chapter Four

THE INFIRMARY WARDS

In 1890 extensions were made on land owned by the Newmarket Workhouse Board of Governors and this seems to have been the provision of the new infirmary buildings in line with the Act of 1867. The infirmary wards consisted of two separate two-storey blocks for male and female patients connected by a main corridor. The buildings used for male patients were the present maternity wards. The pathology department buildings were the original female wards. A block diagram of the new infirmary extensions looked like this:

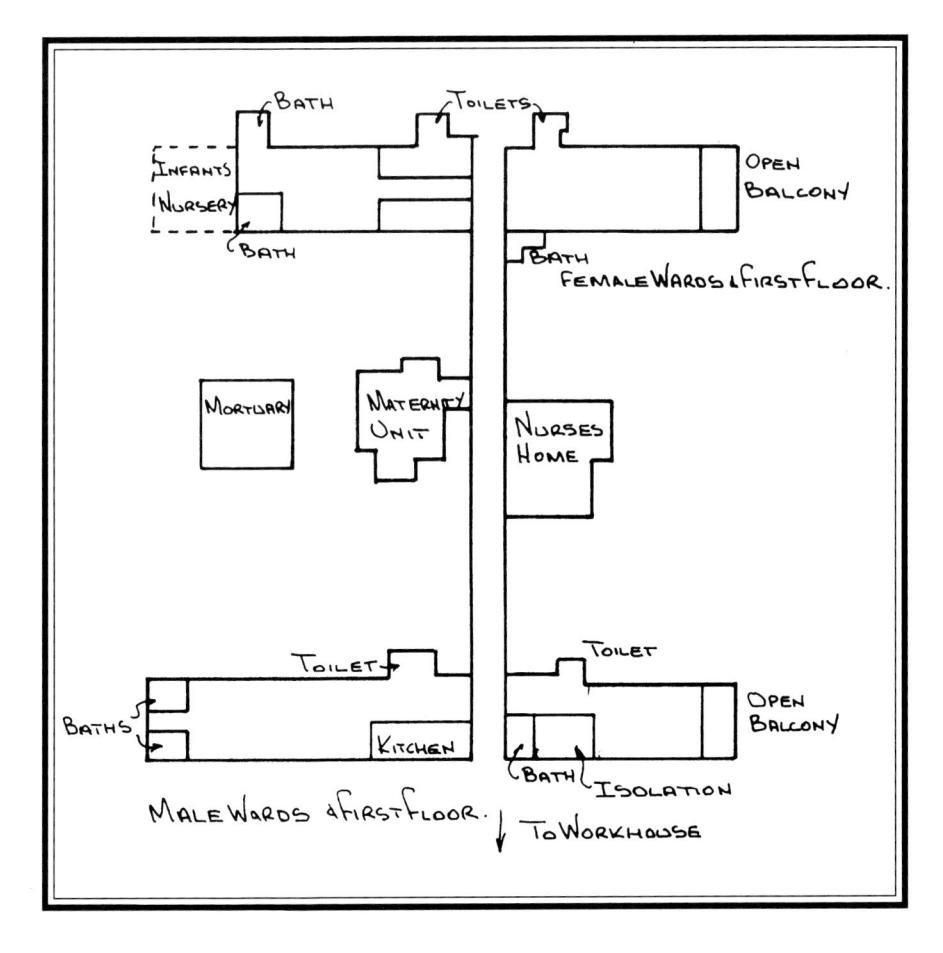

A more detailed block diagram of the complete workhouse/infirmary is shown in the illustrations at page 26. It accommodated about three hundred inmates, both infirm or sick, children and able-bodied whose outdoor relief had been exhausted and who had no work or anywhere to live.

The first local doctors who attended the sick and infirm patients were Dr. Clement Gray, father of Drs. Norman and Gilbert Gray, and Dr. Crompton. Dr. Crompton always wore a black top hat and frock coat and came to the infirmary in a pony and trap. Dr. Maund and, later, Dr. Norman Simpson were the later doctors.

They attended the infirmary wards on three half days a week and would always attend, if needed, in an emergency at any time of the day or night. One day, when a little boy, Dr. Maund told me to open my mouth and he cut off my "uvula". He gave me sixpence for not making a noise: I couldn't with a mouth full of blood.

The eight infirm or sick wards of the infirmary received patients, mainly of a geriatric nature, who could not be nursed at home or could not afford to pay for medical care or were not suitable cases for Addenbrooke's Hospital.

The dispensary was the small room, much later used as the Night Superintendent's Office, medicines were dispensed and issued from here and Dangerous Drugs kept in the special locked cupboard. The Matron was the only qualified person to handle these DDs. She kept the key to the cupboard on her person at all times and was responsible for making up the Dangerous Drugs book. The doctor would see walking cases from the Workhouse here. He did quite a bit of minor surgery and extracted teeth without an anaesthetic.

Epileptic fits were more common in those days and many people became inmates because the fits interfered with their work. It was a common and unpleasant sight to see someone lying on the floor having an epileptic fit. One could only loosen the collar and put something soft under the head and wait for the fit to pass. Although not yet cured it is a relief that medicine has considerably helped this malady today.

The accommodation now used as a "staff creche" opposite the doctors' quarters, was originally built as a Maternity Unit. It was a very active unit and contained "delivery" and "lying in" wards as they were then known. The Matron was the only qualified midwife. She worked long hours and I am sure there are still a number of local people who remember her and the excellent work this unit did for the people of Newmarket.

The mortuary was very primitive and consisted of thick slate slabs fitted into the outside walls with a central table for the occasional post-mortem. It was the duty of the unfortunate porter to assist with post-mortems. There were no facilities for relatives visiting to view the body of an inmate as there are today.

After the infirmary wards were opened definite funeral arrangements were necessary. Although relatives arranged some funerals privately most were arranged by the Institution in public ground at Newmarket Cemetery. It fell to the lot of the Junior Clerk to go by bicycle to Ennion's office to register the death, pay the burial fees, take the order for the grave to be dug to the caretaker of the cemetery and then cycle over to Exning to arrange for the Vicar to take the Service. The hearse was ordered from Messrs. Leader & Griffiths (now the Heath Garage). Four inmates acted as bearers, they were issued with dark suits, black ties and bowler hats kept especially for the purpose and it was the Junior Clerk's job to act as undertaker. I know I did it!

An inmate named Jimmy Gallon was the messenger for the Institution. He posted the mail at the main Post Office and delivered all sorts of things locally.

About 1850 conditions started to improve. Candles were giving way to gas jets. In 1860 Sir Clifford Allbert got a local firm in London to design a thermometer which could be carried in the pocket. This was the start of taking a patient's temperature.

The Board of Guardians

The Workhouse Board of Guardians consisted of local people. A picture of a Mr. Bowcock hung in the Board Room for many years: he must have given excellent service. Later Guardians were Mr. Jimmy Wheeler, who kept the Exning Road post office, Mr. Gurteen from Haverhill, Mr. Troughton, who managed the Gas Works, Mr. Bertie Newton and a Mr. Taylor who always arrived by pony and trap. Their services must have extended well into the early 1930's when the administration of the Workhouse came under the West Suffolk County Council. Major S. J. Ennion, a local solicitor, was the Clerk to the Board of Guardians and his deputy, who attended the Guardians' meetings, was Mr. Blackburn. He was a dapper little man who wore spats and had a waxed moustache. He always carried a neatly rolled umbrella. It was a prank to slide rice or confetti into his umbrella and watch, from a distance, his rather violent reaction when he opened it on a rainy day!

Mr. Boosh Bonham was the managing Clerk at Ennions' offices who dealt with burials and other local routine matters. He moved to Leiston, in Suffolk, and I believe lived happily there for many years.

Mr. A. Charles Guy was the first known Master of the Workhouse, followed by Mr. and Mrs. Vincer Minter in 1889, who were the first Master and Matron. They were highly thought of and a stained glass window, in memory of Mrs. Minter, exists in the church today. My sister tells me her ghost still haunts the Nurses' Training School buildings.

Staff

Early records of 1914 show the following staff in post to administer the Workhouse and nurse the patients in the Infirmary:

Workhouse		Infirmary	
Master	1	Matron	1
Assistant Master	1	Assistant Matron	1
Cook	2	Infants' Attendant	2
Engineer	1	Charge Nurse	2
Laundress	1	Assistant Nurse	4
Needle Mistress	1	Ward Maid	2
Porter/Chargehand	1		

The first recorded member of staff I can find was Mr. Herbert Easter who was the Chargehand Porter from 1889 to 1924. A few others who gave long service were:

George Bedlow	Cook	7 February 1905 to 22 August 1914
Laura Webb	Needle Mistress	12 April 1910 to 16 April 1924
Georgina H. Lockhead	Asst. Nurse	13 November 1912 to 15 December 1934

In 1910 the Needle Mistress was paid a salary of £25 per annum with emoluments valued at £35 per annum. Two references for an unfortunate cook are worthy of note:

> "Ladies and Gentlemen,
>
> I have pleasure in stating that during the three years Mr. A. D. Wiseman has been a cook at this Workhouse he has carried out his duties in a very satisfactory manner. In addition to the routine work in the kitchen, he has regularly relieved the Porters and has assisted generally in other ways. Anything I have asked him to he has done to the best of ability, cheerfully and willingly. I have always found him to be a very quiet, steady, and loyal officer and as such I can with confidence recommend him for the post of Porter for which he is a selected candidate.
>
> I am
>   Yours obediently,
>
> 29.3.1914   Master.

> Dear Sir,
>
> The bearer has been a cook here for 3 years and I have always found him a very decent officer. He could never obtain a Gold Medal for his cooking but I believe he would make a good Porter. He is anxious to get more open air work and appears keen to get to you. I shall be pleased to hear he is successful.
>
>   Yours faithfully,
>
> 29.3.1914.   Master.

At least they were honest in those days! I wonder what the trade unions of today would have said about that poor cook's duties?

The Inmates' Life

The able-bodied inmates of the Workhouse were mainly men and women, some of low mentality. Although most remained inmates permanently some were admitted on a temporary basis and eventually found work or in due course returned to their families. Many sick patients also returned to their homes.

There were three cottages available for families who fell on hard times and were evicted from their homes. They were nearly always issued on a short term basis and were only available to men over the age of 65 years.

Mild forms of witchcraft and spells were much feared in those days and it was not uncommon for an inmate to ply staff with threats of this nature.

Although life for the able-bodied inmates of the Workhouse was far from good, we should remember the essence of charity, both under the Church and the new Guardians, was that people were expected to work for their keep. It was the original intention for the Workhouse to be self-supporting, so far as possible, to keep the demands on the ratepayers low. The able-bodied were required to work in all the productive sections of the Workhouse without payment. Although some were of low mentality , some were tradesmen and educated people whose services were much in demand for work in the Institution. Quite a number of tradesmen passed through tramp wards and were admitted to the Workhouse. More will be said about these people later.

Although no payment was made for work, relatives brought in comforts for the inmates and incentives were given often in the form of 1 oz. of tobacco a week - "SHAG or TWIST". Many people may think that the principle of "Work for Keep" was bad and it did get the Workhouse a bad name. To avoid people being bored in hospitals and institutions today we provide "diversional and occupational therapy" which makes one wonder if they were so wrong years ago!

One ounce of tobacco was also given for every rat caught and it was surprising how effective this method was. The rat tails had to be produced, many smelt badly and it was obvious had been brought up many times before. Those old boys weren't daft! The Assistant Master had to become an expert in detecting fraud.

Mr. Harvey was the foreman gardener whose headquarters was the potting shed. He looked after the greenhouse and supervised the work of the other inmates working on the extensive gardens which produced a variety of excellent flowers, bedding plants and a large quantity of vegetables. Mustard seed was set and dug in the soil to prevent wire worms and to fertilize the ground. I remember the potatoes being raised and put into straw-lined clamps for use in the winter months.

Mr. Harvey was no ordinary person. He presented a fearsome sight. He had a very deep grating voice and an abundance of long black hairs protruding from his ears and nose, these being muddled up with a few warts. He set iron mantraps to keep inmates and others away from the crops and terrified us children, particularly when we climbed his walnut tree.

The woodshed was a main place of work for the men and not only provided firewood for the numerous coke stoves and coal fires in the Institution but was sold to shopkeepers and local people. The trade in firewood was very good and the profit from sales helped to reimburse some of the running costs of the Institution.

Mr. Jim King was the inmate in charge of the woodshed in the early days. He was an old soldier who only had one leg. When the need called, however, he could move at a tremendous speed on a pair of T-shaped crutches.

Tree trunks were purchased, sawn into logs with old cross cut saws. The logs were split with axes and chopped into sticks. Bundling machines were used to tie the sticks into bundles for sale. The firewood was delivered to the shops and houses by a Mr. Jacobs in a picturesque donkey and tub cart which was kept for the purpose. I am sure there are still a few local people who remember them moving about the town.

The Laundry

The hand laundry provided work for female inmates and produced quite a high standard of linen and clothing for the staff, patients and inmates in both the Workhouse and Infirmary. The original laundry looked like the drawing on page 42.

The day to day work in the laundry was supervised by the Laundress and the plant was maintained by the Engineer. The horizontal steam engine was his pride and joy and would be worth a lot of money if it were available today. It was beautifully kept. Its green and red six-foot flywheel always fascinated me as a child. The engine drove the washing machine, hydro-extractor and calender, etc. through a system of shaft-wheels and wide leather belts. A few

The original laundry looked like this.

[Diagram showing laundry layout with labels: Laundry Yard, Hand Lines, Wooden Hand Wash Tubs, Hand Irons, Clean Packing Room, Washing Machine, Steam Engine, Waste Steam Drying Racks, Single Roll Callender, Coke Hand Iron Stove, Very Old Stone Filled Hand Roller Press.]

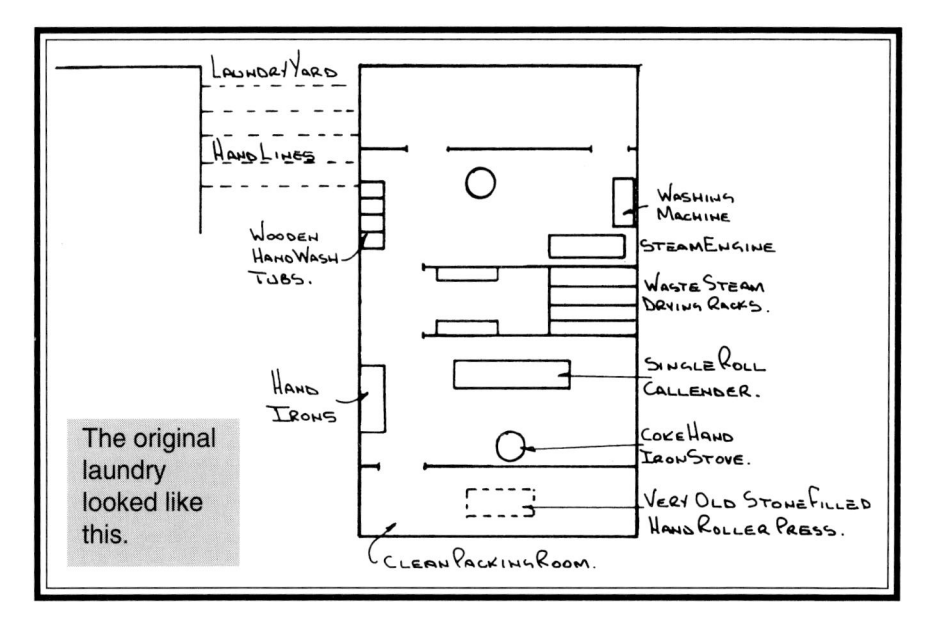

steam-heated drying racks were provided but, whenever the weather permitted, linen was hung out to dry on lines across the laundry yard.

The yard contained a surface water well which provided soft water for the hand wash tubs and washing machine. Another large well was outside the new Nursery or Physiotherapy Department as it is today. They were connected and it was the job of an inmate to hand pump the soft water from the wells to a tank above the drying racks where it was partially heated by steam waste. More will be said later about these wells.

The sewing/linen room played an important role in the day to day life of the Workhouse. It was supervised by the Needle Mistress. Most items of linen were made in the sewing room from large rolls of calico, bleached and unbleached, and other materials. Inmates' and patients' clothing was purchased in bulk and altered to suit individuals. A tight system of marking items was maintained and present staff may find it hard to believe that losses were not tolerated.

Catering

The catering arrangements were simple and effective. The original kitchen and dining room only catered for the inmates of the Workhouse, they were extended to include the new Infirmary wards when they were built. The kitchen was located in "A" Block and was the accommodation later used as Ancillary Staff Changing Rooms, Post/Wages room, etc. There were also two small stores in the basement. The stand-ard of food was pretty cruel: much has already been said about this. There was not much improvement until the responsibilities were transferred to the Local Authorities in 1929. The original layout of the kitchen and dining rooms looked like this:

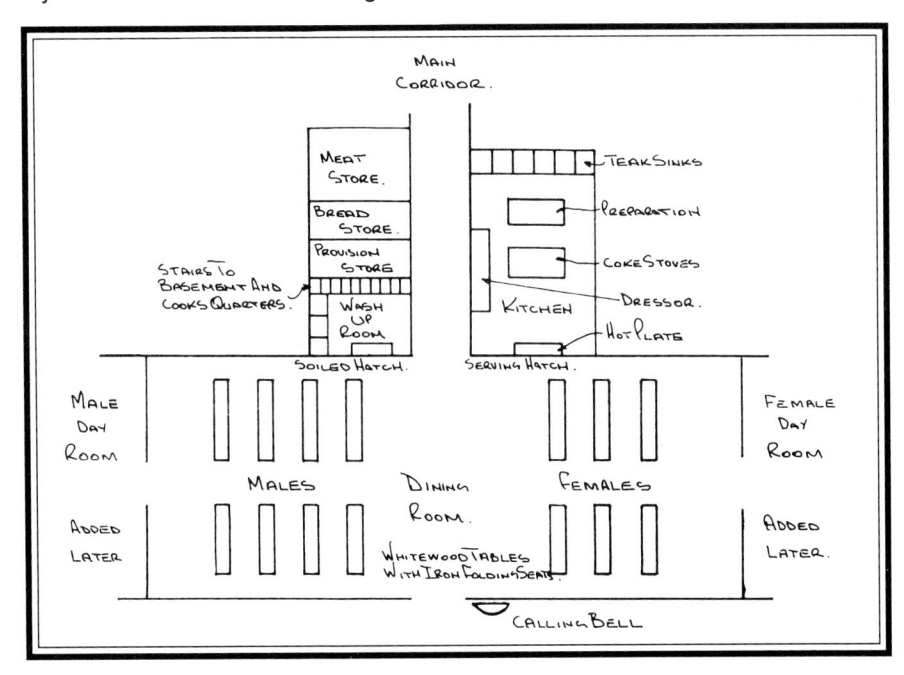

```
                            MAIN
                          CORRIDOR

                    ┌─────────┐     ┌──────────── TEAK SINKS
                    │  MEAT   │     │
                    │  STORE  │     ├──────────── PREPARATION
                    ├─────────┤     │
                    │  BREAD  │     │
                    │  STORE  │     ├──────────── COKE STOVES
   STAIRS TO        ├─────────┤     │
   BASEMENT AND     │PROVISION│     │
   COOKS QUARTERS   │  STORE  │     └──────────── DRESSER
                    ├─────────┤   KITCHEN
                    │  WASH   │           ├────── HOT PLATE
                    │   UP    │
                    │  ROOM   │
                    └─────────┘
                   SOILED HATCH   SERVING HATCH

   MALE          ┌─┐ ┌─┐ ┌─┐ ┌─┐   ┌─┐ ┌─┐ ┌─┐            FEMALE
   DAY           │ │ │ │ │ │ │ │   │ │ │ │ │ │            DAY
   ROOM          └─┘ └─┘ └─┘ └─┘   └─┘ └─┘ └─┘            ROOM
                      MALES        DINING     FEMALES
                                    ROOM
   ADDED         ┌─┐ ┌─┐ ┌─┐ ┌─┐              ┌─┐ ┌─┐ ┌─┐  ADDED
   LATER         │ │ │ │ │ │ │ │              │ │ │ │ │ │  LATER
                 └─┘ └─┘ └─┘ └─┘  WHITEWOOD TABLES └─┘ └─┘ └─┘
                                  WITH IRON FOLDING SEATS
                                         ▽
                                     CALLING BELL
```

My earliest recollection of the kitchen was of an inmate who was the Kitchen Porter. His name was Mr. English and he was reputed to have been a famous jockey when he was young. He had the bandiest legs anyone had ever seen and it was said their shape was caused by fractures due to many falls from race horses. He was a remarkable man: single-handed he hand peeled all the potatoes and prepared the vegetables for the kitchen. He also washed up all the kitchen utensils. He worked hard and long hours for many years and I never heard him complain or of him being off sick.

The able-bodied inmates assembled in the day rooms, attached to the main dining room, and were called to meals by the toll of a bell. It was the duty of the Porter to do this, say Grace at every meal, serve tea, prepare the bread and margarine and generally supervise the arrangements in the dining room. Metal plates and mugs were used and the dirties were handed in to the wash-up hatch by inmates on their way out. After washing-up they were moved back into the main kitchen servery ready for the next meal.

I remember the quick method used for giving the exact weight of margarine. It consisted of a square board with saw cuts around the edges through which a cheese wire was pressed, thus dividing the margarine into exact squares of the correct weight.

The tables and seating arrangements in the dining hall consisted of long combined American White Wood tables and flip up forms. American White Wood is a very clean wood without knots and was scrubbed until it looked really white. Unfortunately they all had to get up at the same time from the seats.

There was little food waste but what there was, was used to feed the pigs and chickens. The pigs were looked after by inmates and for years were slaughtered and cut up by the Prigg family butchers whose shop adjoined the "Cherry Tree" public house in Exning Road. The pork was salted down by the cook and kept on the slate slabs, some being made into brawn and bacon. The pigs' dung was put back into the land as fertilizer and there was no swill to sell as there is today.

Mentally disturbed cases were sent to the Workhouse for assessment and, if necessary, certified insane and sent to the Asylum at Melton near Ipswich. The distance from Newmarket caused untold hardships for relatives wishing to visit a member of their family at Melton. It was a direct result of the unnecessarily silly County boundary and I wonder why people of Newmarket have put up with this inconvenience for so long.

Violent mental cases were put into a straitjacket and then into the padded cell. This was the room, much later, used as a strong room or records room. The porter, cook, Assistant Master or anyone else who could be recruited had to look after these cases until they were sent to Melton. It was the job of the Junior Clerk, with one or two inmates, to accompany the persons to Melton in Mr. Langley's hire car.

Services on the site

Mr. H. Riddington was the first Engineer in memory and the range and amount of work that man did with an old hand pillar drill, comparatively primitive tools and a few nuts and bolts, was quite remarkable. With the assistance of inmates as stokers, occasional tradesmen and general help, he kept all the plant and services going at all costs. He was in charge of the work of the stokers, fitter's shop, blacksmith's shop, carpenter's shop and painters.

The cobbler's and tailor's shops were both essential departments of the Workhouse. The first recorded tailor was a member of the staff named Mr. Lockhead. He repaired and altered the men's suits and clothing: adjustments to ladies' clothing was done in the sewing room.

The cobbler or shoemaker was an inmate who repaired all the inmates' shoes and boots and could be seen hand sewing leather soles with wax ends fitted with bristles to the long threads which he had to make himself. A good shoemaker would also make shoes for the staff by hand. The leather uppers were purchased and he made the rest from very large sheets of leather which were purchased for the repair work.

Two fine horizontal Lancashire Boilers were installed in the boiler house which was adjacent to the original Engineer's shop beneath "A" Block. They provided steam for the laundry and kitchen and limited steam central heating, as well as hot water through a number of hot water calorifiers.

The boilers worked at 60lbs pressure and while one was working the other was closed down for maintenance. It was the job of an inmate, named Dunstal Green because he came from that village, to spend hours inside the boiler and calorifiers to remove the hard lime scale with a special sharp bladed hammer. This had to be done before the Insurance Inspectors came on their annual inspection. Dunstal Green was a hard working lad who used to eat the hard "HEEL" deposit of nicotine from other inmates' pipes. He got a good one one day which knocked him unconscious and flat on his back. He liked playing the mouth organ, rather badly!

I remember, in the late 1920's, a second hand steam donkey pump which fell over and broke its main casting when being installed. It was made of cast iron and was repaired by electrical welding by Messrs. Webbs of Exning and was quite a feat in those days. It gave many years of valuable service after the repair.

One of the earliest stokers was named "Brumey". He worked single handed and came on duty at 7 a.m. and went off duty at 6 p.m. when the main work of the day was over. He had very little off duty time.

The ash from the boiler was carefully kept, watered down and used to damp down the fires at the end of the day. The dampers controlling the air flow to the fires were closed leaving only sufficient air to keep the fires alight. The boilers were left unattended until 7 a.m. next morning but they held sufficient hot water for use during the night.

The Institution had its own water wells: a 100 foot well was located beside the dining hall and supplied most of the Institution's needs. A very old gas engine pumped the water through a system of intermediate pumps and rods to a large tank on the roof above the dining hall. A mention has already been made of other wells used for the laundry. The most interesting was a very deep one found by the carpenter's shop. This was believed to be one of the old ice wells. It was filled with ice in the winter which kept cool for use in the summer months. The Institution was eventually connected to the town water supply.

It has already been mentioned that candles provided lighting for the Institution until about 1850 when gas jets were introduced and used until the town's private "Direct Current" electricity supply was changed to the nationalised "Alternating Current" supply in the early 1930's The gas pipes were old and often filled with water, which dimmed the lights. Telephone calls were often made to Mr. Troughton and, later, Mr. Redfern, managers of the Gas Company, saying "Give us a blow". At this request the gas works staff would clean the filters and blow air through the pipes to remove the water. The jet lights worked much better after this treatment.

Heating throughout the Workhouse and Infirmary was provided by coke fires and although they did not reach the temperatures required in the wards today they were adequate if sufficient coke supplies were available. The coke supplies were often cut to effect economies.

The coke stoves which were installed in the centre of the infirmary wards at a later date were rather unusual. They were about seven feet square and five feet high with perforated grills leading into the ward. Air ducts led under the floor from one outside wall. The chimney duct also ran under the floor to the opposite outside wall. All the heat was kept in the ward and the system was rather like the Baxi fires of today. Gradually the hard-working engineer installed a crude form of central heating into the wards and day rooms. This consisted of long 15 inch diameter cast iron pipes fitted along the skirting boards. Steam at 60lb pressure was fed into one end of the pipe and the other end was fed through the outside wall to a steam trap which released the condensed water. This system was used for many years until someone complained about safety. Reducing steam pressure valves were then fitted in each block building. The system was not half so effective after this. It does show what can be done though.

Security

The security of the Workhouse was very tight. The only entrance was from the Exning Road and the main gates and railings contained iron spikes along their length. The main iron gates were locked at 9 p.m. each night and the key handed into the Porter's Lodge. Staff returning after this time had to ring an outside bell and be let in by the resident porter on duty. They were expected to return by 10 p.m,. at which time the keys were taken to the Master's House. A small wooden hut was located by the entrance and manned by an ex-racing character named Archie. He was on duty from 7 a.m. to 6 p.m. daily and it was his job to enter the name and time of entry and leaving of every person entering the Institution. This book was inspected by the Master each morning.

After receiving a lot of rockets from above for being late in, and following hours of attempted bribery and threats, the engineer agreed to leave one spike on an unseen spring hinge so that the lads did not injure themselves when climbing over the gate in the early hours of the morning.

Two receiving rooms separated by a central bathroom were provided, by the entrance to the Workhouse, for new arrivals who were all required to have a bath. Clean institutional clothing was issued and the inmate's private clothing stored away. The inmate would then pass into the appropriate part of the Workhouse.

All inmates were required to bathe and change their clothing each week. A strict record was kept in the Bath Book which was examined by the Master at regular intervals.

The standard of cleanliness outside was not high and quite a lot of inmates, patients and, particularly, tramps, arrived with lice, vermin and other unwanted lodgers. These were removed from the person when bathed in the receiving rooms. Their clothing was sent to the disinfector before going to the laundry. The disinfector was steam operated and worked at about 20lb steam pressure. It certainly killed all the "naughties" but was very unkind to the clothing, but it had to be done.

Recreation was not very good and was really confined to walking around the grounds in fine weather, playing cards and dominoes in the mens' day rooms and the usual things that ladies do, in the female dayroom. For a number of years, on Saturday afternoons, the ladies put on their best clothes and, under supervision, walked in two ranks down to the Victoria cinema, which was part of the Victoria Hotel, managed by Mr. Lindrum. He very kindly allowed the ladies to see the films free of charge and they certainly appreciated it.

Accommodation was provided for the welfare of destitute children and infants from broken homes. The boys and girls, mainly in the age group of 6 to 12 years were accommodated in the Workhouse. The girls' school and accommodation was that now used as the Nurses Training School in "A" block. The boys were in the end part of the present Admin. block. Although in those days schooling was generally poor, a local school teacher attended regularly and some form of education was given. This was not always the case outside. Most of the girls were eventually found work in service and the boys would work on farms or as apprentices to trades.

Chapter Five

THE CASUAL WARDS

Vagrancy has always been a problem and remains so today although we now call it something else and deal with it in a different way.

Part of the Gilbert Act of 1782 made it compulsory for wards to be provided *"..for the Casual Stay of Gentlemen and Ladies of the Road passing through the towns."* The male casual wards at Newmarket were built as part of and run by the Workhouse. They were located, adjoining Exning Road, and were on the left of the present entrance to the hospital It later became the A.R.P. centre during World War 2.

The female casual ward was located near the hospital Church and was a building at the end of the inmates' married accommodation and formed the boundary wall with the Exning Road Working Mens' Club. When first built all the land between the Workhouse and Bakers Row was open fields.

A sketch of how the original casual ward was laid out is as under:

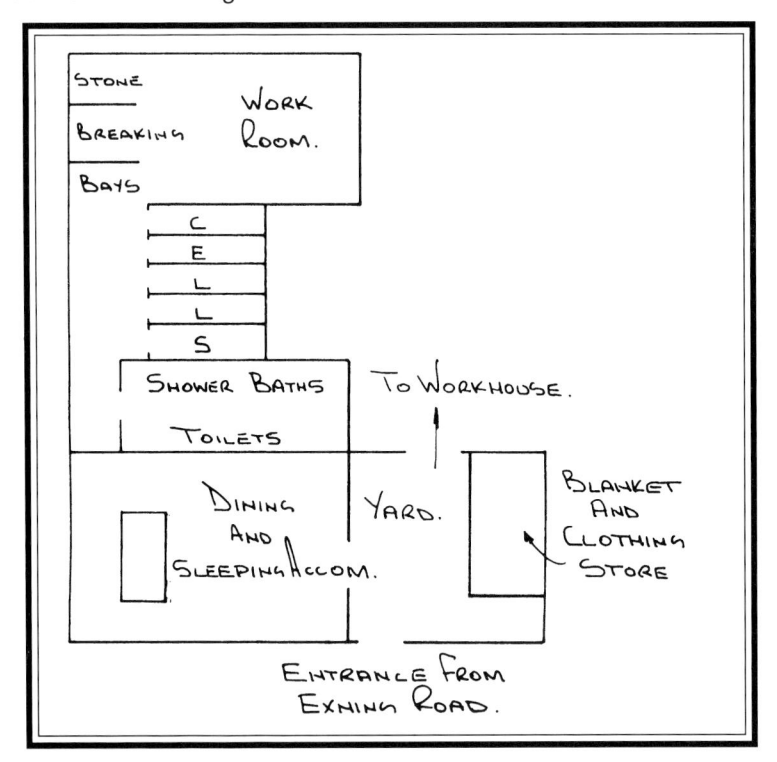

```
┌─────────────────────────────────────────────┐
│ ┌──────────────────────────┐                │
│ │ STONE                    │                │
│ │ ─────       WORK         │                │
│ │ BREAKING    ROOM.        │                │
│ │ BAYS                     │                │
│ │      ┌───────┐           │                │
│ │      │  C    │           │                │
│ │      ├───────┤           │                │
│ │      │  E    │           │                │
│ │      ├───────┤           │                │
│ │      │  L    │           │                │
│ │      ├───────┤           │                │
│ │      │  L    │           │                │
│ │      ├───────┤           │                │
│ │      │  S    │           │                │
│ │      └───────┘           │                │
│ ├──────────────────┐       │                │
│ │ SHOWER BATHS     │ TO WORKHOUSE.          │
│ │ ┌─────┐          │       ↑                │
│ │ │TOILETS│        │       │                │
│ └─┴─────┴──────────┘       │   ┌──────────┐ │
│                            │   │ BLANKET  │ │
│   ┌───┐ DINING   YARD.     │   │   AND    │ │
│   │   │  AND               │   │ CLOTHING │ │
│   │   │ SLEEPING ACCOM.    │   │  STORE   │ │
│   └───┘                    │   └──────────┘ │
│                                              │
│              ENTRANCE FROM                  │
│              EXNING ROAD.                   │
└─────────────────────────────────────────────┘
```

Other casual wards were built as part of the Workhouses at Cambridge, Linton, Bury St. Edmunds, Haverhill, Sudbury, and all the other towns of any size. A day's tramp was about fourteen miles but the more experienced casuals would often walk at least twenty-eight miles to avoid a particular ward which had a bad reputation for hospitality.

The gentlemen of the road, or tramps as they were then known, tramped the length and breadth of the county. To many it was a way of life but others were honestly looking for work and followed the seasons. They came to East Anglia for work on the land and for the harvest and sugar beet picking. A lot were drawn to Newmarket for the horse racing. They went to Kent for the hop and soft fruit picking and to all the other counties where casual work was available.

During the summer months many slept rough in woods or hedgerows and only came into the casual wards when they needed food or as a hygienic necessity. At one time as many as thirty tramps were admitted to the casual ward in one night and conditions were made very bad, but within the law, to discourage them from coming to Newmarket. It was remarkable how quickly the word was passed on and the numbers reduced considerably.

Although most tramps were reasonable people, unfortunately, some of them were drunks and undesirables who caused endless trouble for the limited staff who had to deal with them.

The casual wards were open for admissions from 6 p.m. to 9 p.m. on Monday to Saturday. On arrival the usual particulars were taken, viz name, age, occupation, domiciliary, where they came from and their destination. The admission orders were examined by the Master the following day and it was surprising how well the habits, good and bad, of the habitual callers were known. Newcomers were picked out and often helped.

It was the rule that tramps should pay for their keep if they had money. They were searched and any valuables, offensive weapons, methylated spirits, alcohol, etc. confiscated and the good things returned when they were discharged two days later. It became well known that tramps packed up their money, valuables and other items and hid them in hedges and other places before they went into the tramp wards. They would pick them up again when discharged.

Fred Coleman, whose family kept the "Cherry Tree" for many years told some wonderful tales about the tricks the tramps used to get up to. Unfortunately he is now no longer with us.

Tramps had to work the day following admission and this took many forms, such as breaking up stones for concrete, chopping wood, sweeping the grounds, teasing out coir fibre for remaking mattresses, etc.

In 1933 at the age of seventeen, my brother Reg tramped the road for a week accompanied by an old tramp. He was interested in the life of a tramp and did this to gain experience.

On arrival all tramps were issued with clean blankets and night attire and compelled to have a hot bath under the supervision of the porter. They were given a hot meal consisting of a pint of tea, 6 oz. bread and 2 ozs. margarine, together with something hot. Normal meals were issued the next day.

A mention has been made of the ability of some of the tramps passing through the casual wards and much more will be said in the next chapter. In the original dining room, later known as the Blue Room, four very large oil paintings were painted directly on to the walls. They were about nine feet by five feet in size and were painted in about 1920 by a tramp named Mr. Grace. They were admired by many people for many years and it was a shame that wear and tear made it necessary to paint over them when the room was redecorated.

A picture of the front of the Workhouse, as it was in 1927, is shown on the following page. It was painted by a tramp named James Wanless. The Austin 7 car belonged to the Relieving Officer, who, I am pretty sure, was Mr. W. B. Hatley.

The original painting, appropriately framed, now hangs in the main entrance of the new Hospital.

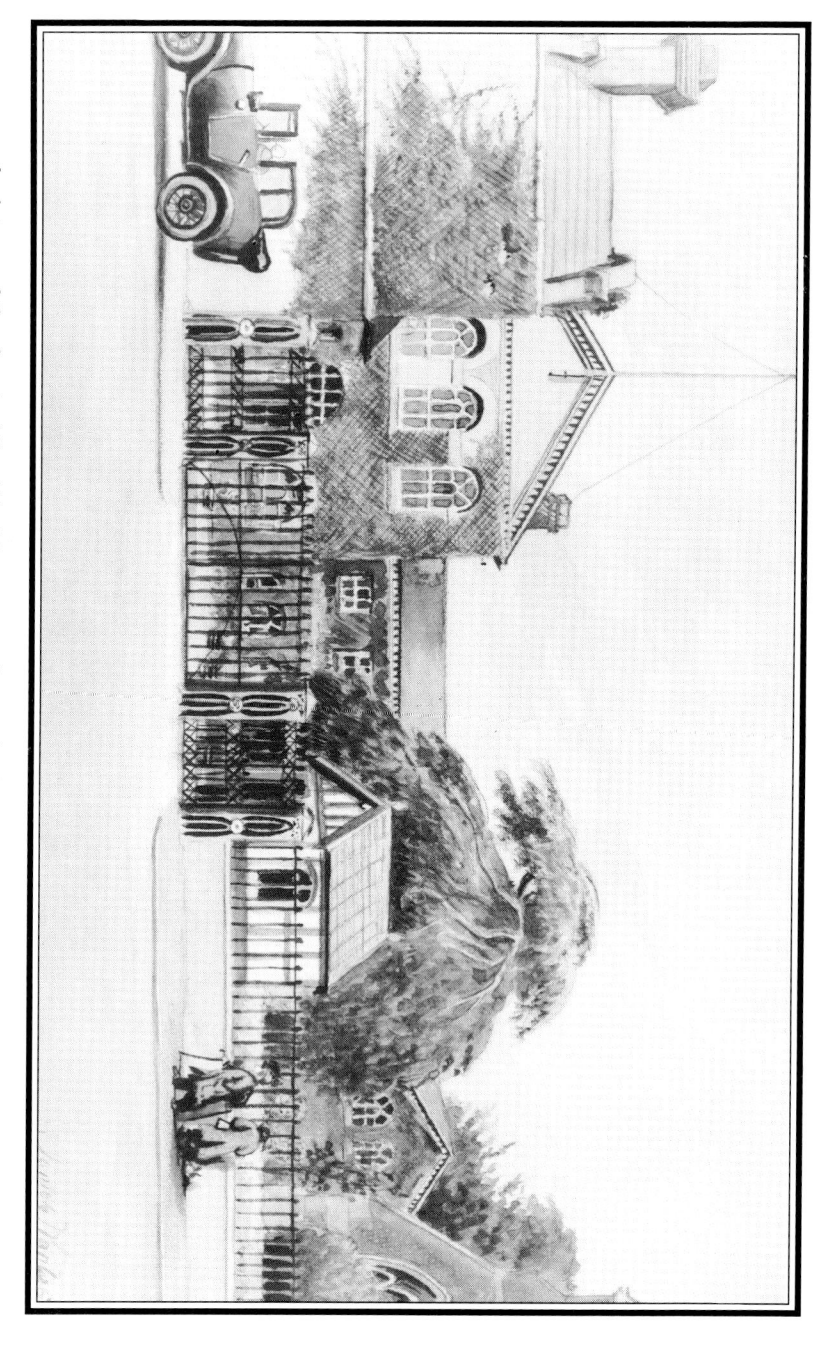

A picture of the front of the Workhouse, as it was in 1927, painted by James Wanless.

52

Chapter Six

THE PUBLIC ASSISTANCE INSTITUTION

In 1929 the new Public Assistance Act put the responsibility for the relief of the poor and sick squarely on the shoulders of the County Councils. The Act was introduced in 1930.

The 1930's saw the Workhouses changed into the Public Assistance Institutions, working alongside the voluntary hospitals. The involvement of the County Councils made them responsible for all the Institutions and primary care within their county and they were able to coordinate the work and resources as the need required. The day to day work of the Institution was still left in the hands of the Master and Matron.

The work of the local doctors remained outside the new system. In 1930 the excellent services previously carried out by Major S. J. Ennion and his staff were transferred to the West Suffolk County Council in Bury St. Edmunds.

A central system of funding was set up under the control of Mr. Sayers, the County Accountant, and this led the way to a much more flexible service. Mr. Hinnel did most of the public assistance work for his department and he was a very good friend to Newmarket. Mr. Hazelton, who played rugby for Bury St. Edmunds and told very rude jokes, was the internal auditor.

Mr. Munsey was the Clerk of the West Suffolk County Council and a small Public Assistance Sub Section was added to his department. Mr. Freddie Thompson was appointed Public Assistance Officer and it was his duty to coordinate the work of the Institutions and the new Relieving Officers for both indoor and outdoor relief throughout the county. John Crease was the County Architect and Dr. Rogers was the County Medical Officer of Health. Later this appointment was held by Dr. MacCracken with Dr. Rae as his deputy. Mr. White was responsible for the public assistance administration work of the CMO department. These were excellent officers and much is owed for their help and guidance.

The Board of Guardians were dissolved and House Committees were appointed. Again the members were local business men. The names of two well known members were Captain H. R. King and Mr. Bertie Newton.

For those in need of relief

A word should be said about the system of "outdoor relief" which was set up for local people needing help.

The Relieving Officers had wide powers and could act without reference to committee or without a lot of paper work. They did, however, report to a small sub-committee who met quarterly. I believe this was more a progress and endorsement committee.

It was the Police, District Nurse, the Vicar, local Doctor or any member of the public who drew the attention of the Relieving Officer to the plight of a person needing help. He would visit the person's house without delay and make an assessment. If admission to the Infirmary or Workhouse was necessary he would arrange the admission and transport on the spot. In urgent cases the Relieving Officer could arrange admission to another Institution if a bed was not available locally.

For people needing outdoor relief, the Relieving Officer would, where he thought fit, give orders direct to local traders for supplies of groceries, meat, coal and other listed necessities to be delivered direct to the person's house. Some money was given but only for essentials. It made sure people were fed, clothed and kept warm. Money could not be spent on beer and other pleasures as it is today.

Mr. W. B. Hatley was the Relieving Officer for Exning and Newmarket and Mr. Hall for the Haverhill area. Mr. Pearmain covered the Mildenhall district and was succeeded by Mr. J. O. Wiggin, who is still a local councillor for the Mildenhall district.

During the 1930's there was a general feeling of improvement and Masters were encouraged by the County Council to upgrade the conditions and services in the Institutions. Mr. and Mrs. Ernest S. Heasman were the Master and Matron at Newmarket and the hospital owes much to their foresight and drive in the early days in upgrading the Institution to such a state that led to its eventual selection and conversion into a large Emergency Medical Service (E.M.S.) Hospital of nearly 1,000 beds during the 1939-1945 War years.

Using their skills

Only limited funds were available and the engagement of outside contractors was not always possible. The services of skilled tradesmen and labour had to be found elsewhere. A mention has already been made of the number of skilled tradesmen and other professional people passing through the casual wards: these skills were recruited whenever possible.

Selected tramps passing through the town were offered a long stay in the Institution in return for their keep and a small wage. They lived separately from the inmates in the inmates' married accommodation which had been converted for the purpose and were free to come and go as they pleased outside of working hours. Some stayed for a week or two and then were found missing one morning. Some were grateful for the opportunity to sort out their lives and stayed for two or three years. But as always when the sun began to shine their feet began to itch and one day they would be gone. However, many were first class tradesmen and did excellent work for the Institution during their comparatively short stay.

Two excellent carpenters were a Mr. Allard and a Mr. Coston. They built the large wooden nursery which, much later, became the Physiotherapy Department. They also laid and repaired most of the wood block flooring throughout the Institution and repaired the furniture and did all the other work carpenters do. Mr. Moleneux, a first class cabinet maker, stayed for quite some time and some of his work must still be about today. It was nice to see him match the grains of the wood before starting work.

Other tradesmen who stayed were bricklayers, stokers, fitters, blacksmiths, shoemakers, painters, etc.

The type of upgrading work which was done during the 1930's, mostly with the help of these tradesmen, was:

(a) installation of electric lighting and power and all the consequent developments.

(b) the building of the new nursery which has already been mentioned.

(c) the first floor of the Workhouse buildings were open roofed. Ceilings were fitted and the accommodation generally upgraded.

(d) new toilet and bathing facilities were built on to the able-bodied inmates' accommodation.

(e) new wood block floors were laid in the wards, day room and dining rooms.

(f) improved steam heating was installed throughout.

(g) improved laundry facilities - hand washing tubs were replaced by washing machines. Hydro extractors were fitted.

(h) improved kitchen facilities - extra steam boilers and improved cooking stoves fitted. The first refrigerator was installed in the late 1930's, quarry tile floors were laid.

(i) the replacement of the old iron windows in the able-bodied inmates' accommodation with wooden windows was programmed. I believe a few of the iron type still remain today.

(j) curtains were fitted and the wards and buildings redecorated both inside and out. The accommodation was made much more pleasant to live in.

There were many other improvements made in the 1930's. With the upgrading going on more interest was taken by both patients, inmates and staff.

The able-bodied inmates were issued with 1 oz. tobacco each week and the ladies were given sweets. The weekly trips to the cinema continued and local Concert Parties often gave performances which were very much enjoyed. The Post Office always gave a good concert. The Newmarket Town Band played a selection of carols on Christmas morning and visits were always made by local Church Choirs at Christmas-time.

The "Cherry Tree" public house became more popular!

The feeding arrangements were considerably improved. A two week and, later, a three week, cycle menu was introduced and the food generally became much more interesting. There was still very little waste because the exact numbers to be fed were known and I well remember that the lads in the office would fight, in a pleasant way, the porters for the left overs of three pieces of treacle duff and one pint of meat stew. It was jolly good and all that was left over after feeding about two hundred people.

The Institution staff worked hard and long hours and I well remember as the office boy it was one of my many duties to issue the ingredients to the cook for the meal the following day. This had to be done between 4 and 4.30 p.m. and was doubled up at weekends. Quantities were worked out on fixed scales. A long, very accurate, Blue Book was used. A page was reserved for each dish. The ingredients required were listed down the left hand side of the page and the number of people to be fed was listed across the top. It was a simple matter to read off the ingredients and amounts required for each dish. It was also my duty to issue provisions such as jam, sugar, tea and general groceries to the Nurses' Home and other staff quarters between 12.30 and 1 p.m. on Saturday mornings each week.

The names of some old-time members of the staff have been mentioned. A few others were two sisters, Miss Violet and Miss Ethel Lambert, who were the Assistant Matron and Laundress between 1925 and 1941. Violet was killed in an air raid on Newmarket on 18th February, 1941. Mr. Frank Thomas, Mr. N. E. Kendall and Mr. Frank Page were Assistant Masters and it was nice that Mr. Kendall returned to the hospital, as Group Supplies Officer, when the National Health Service was formed in 1948. Mr. H. Wright and Mr. Robert Pritchard were the porters up to 1936. They were replaced by the Kaye brothers who remained in post up to the War. Nurse E. Rahill was the Qualified Charge Nurse up to 1940.

Although life in the Newmarket Public Assistance Institution became much more active in the 1930's there was little change in its nature. The County Council made other arrangements for the care and teaching of children and the new nursery became a County Centre for the Infants. Many infants were adopted or went home and it was very nice that some returned, when grown up, to thank the staff and let them know how they had progressed.

Inspection

The Department of Health set up a system of Inspectors who made random inspections of all Institutions. The Inspectors were well trained and powerful people. They arrived without notice and the Master was personally responsible for implementing their recommendations. Woe betide the Master who had not acted by the time of their next visit! In a way they were rather like the General Nursing Council's Inspectors who still remain today. Their visits were shorter and reports much more direct.

I remember an Inspector instructing that all lavatory chains should be replaced by rods. The chains had been used by some patients elsewhere to commit suicide and the rods were installed in a very short time in all the Institutions throughout the country.

If the Inspector system applied today I feel a much more uniform service would result without the multitude of committees and duplicated layers of administration.

In 1933 the accommodation in "A" block, vacated by the boys' school, was let as office accommodation to the Newmarket Rural District Council. They eventually moved to their new offices in Park Lane. The accommodation vacated by the girls' school became the Master's and Matron's residential accommodation.

Although our work was not connected in any way, I have pleasant memories of the association with the Newmarket Rural District Council. Mr. Tom Brown was the Clerk of the Council and Sid Marshall and Bert Mingay were members of his staff. Dear old Frank Tomlinson was the Surveyor and the arrival of his first motor car "Myrtle I" was the envy of us all. Frank was rather a large person, in fact, he was very large, too large to fit into "Myrtle's" driving seat so he had a kind of armchair fitted, which made us all sympathise with "Myrtle". These are only some of the RDC staff I remember.

One day my wicked brother substituted the daily tea pint of milk for the Public Health Section with flour and water. He stirred it well all the way to the office and left rather quickly. There was quite a long delay before a very serious young Assistant Sanitary Inspector, Mr. Hawkins, arrived and demanded to know who supplied the milk because his tests had proved, beyond doubt, that the cow had a diseased udder! Evasive action was taken and the matter reported with some vigour to Tom Brown. The rest of the story is left to your imagination: they were happy days!

In late 1938 war clouds were gathering and the Newmarket Public Assistance Institution was visited by two gentlemen from the Ministry of Health. They made a long and thorough inspection of the buildings and the adjoining paddocks. We did not know then that the Institution had been selected as one of the large Emergency Medical Service Hospitals to be built in East Anglia for casualties in the event of war being declared.

Chapter Seven

WHITE LODGE EMERGENCY HOSPITAL
THE WAR YEARS

1939 *The Emergency Medical Service*

When war was declared in 1939 the Ministry of Health set up the Emergency Medical Services (EMS) to cope with the vast number of service personnel and casualties to be expected in a war. This included the Emergency Hospitals. By September 1940 the War Office had published a memorandum listing all the types of hospitals available and the arrangements for admission and the reception of sick and wounded from overseas.

East Anglia quickly became a densely populated area for training the Army, Air Force and other Services and the Newmarket Public Assistance Institution was nominated to be upgraded and developed to serve the area as one of the large Emergency Hospitals containing just under 1,000 beds.

The Ministry of Health set up a small team of experts to design the EMS and the hospitals in it. It became obvious that a great deal of work had already been done before we declared war on Germany because items of inventory were arriving at the hospital before any bricks for the extensions had been laid. Orders had been placed centrally and the staff establishments and building designs decided without the encumbrance of the never ending consultations and the Committee structures which we have to endure today.

The EMS hospitals were designed for speed of construction and contained only the essential facilities. They were only expected to last for ten years and to avoid construction delays whatever local materials were available were used.

The services were situated at one end of the ward alongside the main corridor and were easily accessible for servicing. The disadvantage was the distance the staff and patients had to walk from the far end of the ward to the toilets, baths and other services.

The constant stream of equipment arriving for the new hospital made life very difficult and confusion reigned for some time. The difficulties were exacerbated because Mr. E. S. Heasman, who was still the Master, with foresight, had purchased large quantities of provisions which proved invaluable as the war progressed and rationing was introduced. They were stored in the pig sties, up chimneys and anywhere out of the rain and out of the view of visiting

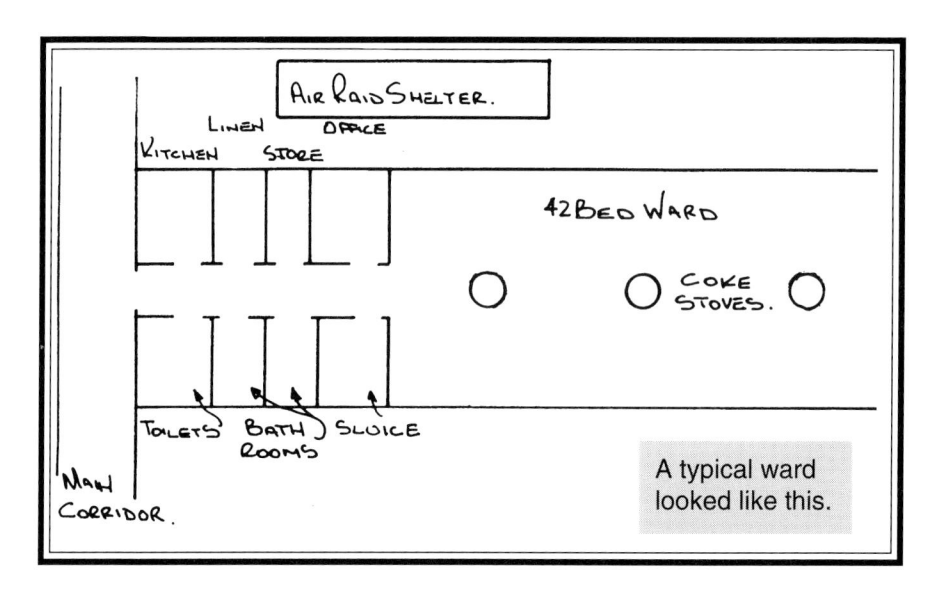

```
           ┌─────────────────┐
           │ Air Raid Shelter.│
     Linen  └──Office─────────┘
    Kitchen    Store
  ┌────────────────────────────────────────────
  │ ┌─┐┌─┐┌─┐┌─┐
  │ │ ││ ││ ││ │           42 Bed Ward
  │
  │                     O         O Coke    O
  │ ┌─┐┌─┐┌─┐┌─┐                    Stoves.
  │ │ ││ ││ ││ │
  │
  │    Toilets  Bath   Sluice
  │            Rooms
   Main
   Corridor.
```
A typical ward looked like this.

Auditors! He received many rockets for this dreadful act but the provisions were very much appreciated and were much in demand as the war progressed.

To add to the confusion, about this time a large blue Packhard car arrived containing Mr. J. Rowlands, who was an excellent surgeon and a very nice chap, together with Sister Kingswell, who was to be in charge of the new theatres, with two Ward Sisters Shepherd and Robinson. They had been directed to the hospital by the Ministry of Health and really were the start of the EMS Hospital. Shortly afterwards Colonel Watson arrived to be Medical Superintendent and Miss Lithgow to be the new Matron.

At the outbreak of war the young men were conscripted into the forces and the young ladies and men unsuitable for active service and in reserved occupations were directed by the Ministry of Labour and Health Service to work in the hospitals, munition factories and other essential services for the war effort. This meant there was no difficulty in staffing the hospitals during the war years but when hostilities ceased and people returned to their homes and jobs the hospitals were left well understaffed with serious consequences. More will be said about this difficulty later.

I remember the strong belief, shared by most people at the time, that the Germans had no chance of breaking through the Maginot Line and that we had thousands of aeroplanes in store at Duxford which were being prepared to sort out the Germans. We really thought the Germans could not hold out for more than six months and someone wrote a song entitled "We're going to hang out our washing on the Siegfried Line". After the evacuation of Dunkirk the song went out of fashion and it was realised what horror our politicians had led the British people into.

In September 1939 the Public Assistance Institution contained 235 inmates and during that month 147 tramps had passed through the casual wards. These wards were closed in October 1939 and it is interesting that in January 1940 Mr. A. F. Langley of the Temperance Hotel in Market Street was paid £10 per annum to issue Vagrancy tickets to tramps seeking accommodation in Newmarket.

1940 *A difficult year*

By September 1940 all the original accommodation was available for EMS use and contained 103 service patients and 4 civilian patients. The name was then changed to "White Lodge Emergency Hospital."

The first air raids started in April and many casualties were admitted following the evacuation of the British Expeditionary Force from Dunkirk which took place between 27th May and 3rd June. The W.R.V.S. and A.R.P. services were called in to help with transport, documentation, feeding, etc. They did wonderful work and their services were invaluable throughout the war years.

There is no doubt that 1940 and 1941 were the most difficult years. Service patients were being admitted at an ever increasing rate at the same time as the accommodation was being changed into a modern Emergency General Hospital. The original Institution buildings were named "A" Block and at the end of 1939 work started on building six new EMS type wards on existing garden land. The wards added 252 beds to the complement and was known as "B" Block.

In July the dining room in "A" Block was divided to form an Outpatient Department with a through corridor for access to the main hospital. In this month it was decided that a further nine wards were required to provide a further 360 beds, together with essential new departments: X-ray, theatres, main kitchens, mortuary, stores and a new boiler house and plant etc. For this purpose 1½ acres of Major Beaty's paddocks were requisitioned and the new site was named "C" Block.

Major Beaty did not like the idea of losing his land and used the most dreadful language to anyone within hearing range.

By October the original inmates' house accommodation in "A" Block had been divided by curtains to provide a crude form of cubicle accommodation for 57 nurses and sisters who had been directed to work in the hospital. The room in "A" Block, recently used as a Sisters' Changing Room, was made into a temporary X-ray Department and a new American Deans X-Ray Set was installed. The offices opposite were then used as changing rooms.

On 4th October it was agreed that the day to day management of the hospital should continue under the Sub-committee of the Public Assistance Department of the West Suffolk County Council as agent of the Ministry of Health in Cambridge. Their services were essential.

At the same meeting it was reported that sixty mothers and children had been admitted to the hospital on the 1st and 3rd October, 1940, for a rest. They were part of the National Evacuation Scheme and were moving from London to parts of Suffolk.

In November the entrance hut, iron gates and railings were removed and melted down to make bombs like those of everyone else. The tub pony cart, now surplus to requirements, was transferred to Sudbury Public Assistance Institution.

The staff in post were:

Administration	Officers` Servants	12 -average salary £65 p.a. 23 -wage £2.l0s.0d.per week, 14s.0d. per week deducted from wage if resident.
Medical Staff	Colonel Watson Professor Maxwell Mr. J. Rowlands Dr. Arden Jones Dr. J. Arnott Dr. F. R. Berridge (part-time)	Miss D. Lawrence appointed as Medical Superintendent's Clerk in September, 1940
Radiographer	Miss D. Cullen	Mrs. V. Berridge (part-time)

Assistants	Miss Ruth Hobbs
	Miss Vogel
Masseurs	Mrs. Thompson
	Miss V. Haytor
Dispenser	Mr. G. H. Burdon

At the December meeting it was reported:

(a) twelve pigs were ready for market.

(b) emergency field cooking apparatus was now available at Newmarket and Bury St. Edmunds to be operated by II Corps DDDM in emergencies.

(c) The services of Mr. Humphries as chimney sweep be retained at a cost of 1s. 6d. per chimney.

(d) a covered way between the new "B" Block and the old "A" Block would be required for the protection of patients.

(e) a battery-type emergency lighting set and 24 hurricane lamps had been purchased for the theatre.

(f) the following quotations for coke supplies had been received:

Newmarket Gas Co.	£2. 11s. 4d. per ton
Southwold Gas Co.	£2. 13s. 10d. per ton
Leiston Gas Co.	£2. 9s. 6d. per ton

(g) the B.R.C.S. had allocated an operating table to the hospital.

(h) Lady Butler had kindly presented the hospital with a headphone wireless set installation.

1941 *The Hospital at War*

On 18th February Newmarket High Street was bombed. Seven people died including Miss V. Lambert and Miss Peck who were members of the hospital staff. A large increase in civilian casualties resulted and some troops had to be transferred to other hospitals to make room for them.

By March the tramp wards had been converted into an A.R.P. and decontamination centre. Miss Marriott was in charge of the First Aid Post.

The six new wards in "B" Block had been opened in February and thus relieved the pressure for beds in "A" Block.

The layout of "B" Block looked like this:

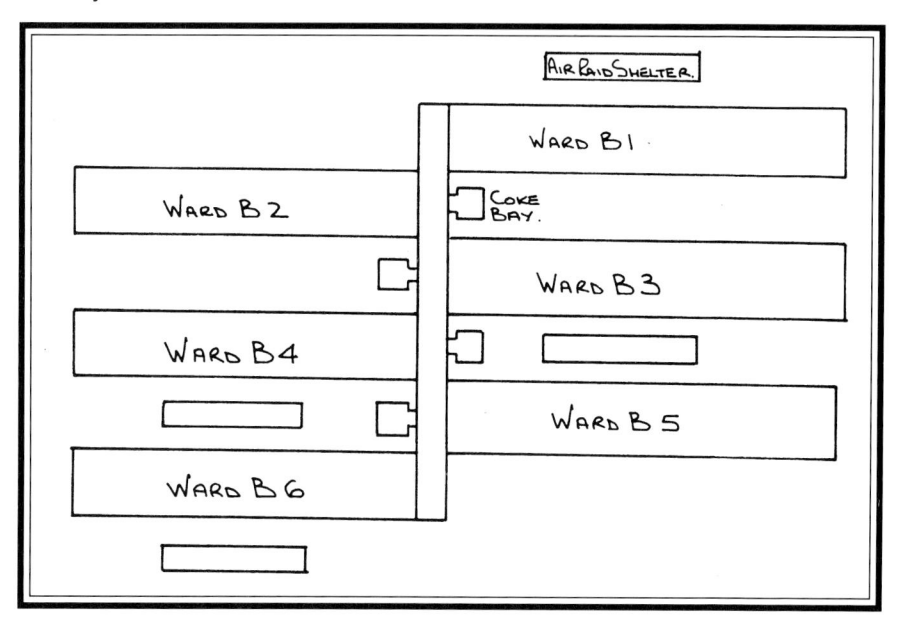

[Diagram of "B" Block layout showing: Air Raid Shelter, Ward B1, Ward B2, Coke Bay, Ward B3, Ward B4, Ward B5, Ward B6]

In April Edward Ward, which was opposite the temporary theatre in "A" Block, was converted into a Resuscitation Room.

At this time there were four Quaker orderlies working in the hospital. The members of the administrative staff working in the Master's Office were Miss P. Fisher, Gordon Carter and Peter Gould and I am sure many people will remember Miss Gibbons who worked in the Nurses' Home for many years and was a much respected member of the staff.

By May the children had been sent elsewhere and the nursery was then used as a Massage and Physiotherapy Department. It proved ideal for the purpose and is still used as such today. Male tuberculosis patients were accommodated in the open balcony of this department in 1942.

On 9th May, a team from the Ministry of Health visited the hospital to check progress and agree further developments. A large steam operated drum sterilizer was to be provided for "C" Block to replace the outdated dangerous gas operated one.

In June the day room on the ground floor of the former female infirmary in "A" Block was converted into an extension to the Pathology Department which was on the first floor above. Dr. Murray was appointed Pathologist on 4th August.

Fire watchers, in the event of air raids, were recruited from the staff and Major Albury was appointed Group Military Registrar for the Cambridge Group.

Dr. Morton Gill had joined the staff. He specialized in Gastric Analysis, etc. and introduced the gastroscope to this service. I was told that some troops were given a pint of beer if they swallowed the thing: what some people will do for a pint!

By October Army manoeuvres were more active and the hospital became much busier. Mr. Rowlands was in charge of all fracture cases which were grouped in Ward A3. Later that year Mr. Jasper Bonnin took over orthopaedic surgery which allowed Mr. Rowlands to concentrate on general surgery.

Messrs. Kings of Exning started building a new pack store for service patients' clothing and a new mortuary in "C" Block and at long last electric power and light was installed in the laundry. As late as August, 1942 it was reported that the coke stove in the laundry was cracked and the hand flat irons which it heated were dirty.

The Enquiry office and telephone kiosk were built in the entrance hall in "A" Block. Telephones were strictly controlled by the Ministry of Health and they agreed that a new switchboard and fourteen additional extensions should be provided, some of which were for the new "C" Block. Miss Ashman was appointed telephonist for which she was paid the princely sum of 10d. per hour.

A storm in the late autumn of 1941 flooded the new "B" Block wards and they were subject to this flooding until the corridor was enclosed some years later. Often staff had to be called back to the hospital to bale the water out of the wards with buckets. In a bad storm six inches of water flooded Wards B5 and B6 and lockers and other furniture could be seen floating about.

On 4th December thirty-nine evacuee children arrived at the hospital unexpectedly and all sorts of funny arrangements had to be made to accommodate them. An increasing number of nursing staff were being directed to the hospital by the Ministry of Health and extra nurses' accommodation was needed. The rooms above the administrative offices in "A" Block were turned into rooms for nursing orderlies and "Cleveland House" in Newmarket was requisitioned and turned into a home to accommodate twenty-five nurses.

1942 *The Hospital developing*

On 17th February Mrs. A. V. Heasman, who had been Matron of the Infirmary and Public Assistance Institution for the past thirty years, retired owing to ill health. Mr. E. S. Heasman was appointed Clerk and Steward for the administration of the new EMS Hospital and the last traces of the Workhouse and Public Assistance Institution had gone. The Institution had done wonderful work during the 106 years since it was first built in 1836.

It was noted that the local 2 Corps Canteen Committee had sent 200lbs of geese to the hospital for Christmas and that the manager of the Doric Cinema had made twenty seats available, free, for the use of service patients.

Between 1941 and 1942 Dr. Arden Jones recruited a number of medical staff from the West London Teaching Hospital in Hammersmith. They included Dr. Morton Gill (orthopaedic), Mr. J. Grant Bonnin (orthopaedic), Dr. M. Welply (house surgeon) and Dr. J. M. Platts (house physician). Dr. Bobby Hall White, a Harley Street physician, was recruited by Professor Ryle, the Regius Professor of Medicine to Cambridge University.

During 1942 the hospital developed rapidly. In February "C" Block was opened and the number of available beds increased to 700. In March, the X-ray Department was moved to the new accommodation in "C" Block and the old room in "A" Block was used as a store.

The Ministry of Health requested a ward to be set aside for children. Part of the ground floor in A3 ward was used for this purpose.

The surgical cases in "A" and "B" Blocks were transferred to wards near the new theatres in "C" Block. The ward vacated in "A" Block was used for tuberculosis patients.

On 20th February Miss M. Welply was appointed orthopaedic house surgeon and Mr. G. Thompson was appointed Pharmacist. They were both solid members of the staff and did excellent work.

On 5th March the Admiralty gave instructions that nineteen sailors from H.M.S. Worcester were to be given one pint of beer daily - some were lucky!

On 26th March the Occupational Therapy and Remedial Medicine Department was opened and a P.T. Instructor was appointed.

Air raids on Norwich took place in April and to make room for casualties from the Norwich area 175 patients were admitted to White Lodge EMS from the Norfolk & Norwich and Woodlands Hospitals. The more seriously injured or sick were admitted and the others moved on to the Three Counties Hospital, Bedford.

The members of the Hospital Committee in May 1942, were Mr. J. B. Coster (Chairman), Mrs. Stafford Allen, Mr. W. H. Hunt, Mr. B. Newton, Mrs. F. W. Ramsey and Mr. J. Wheeler.

The total patients numbered 551. Of these 36 were civilians and one was an evacuee. The staff numbered 395: 15 doctors, 216 nurses and 164 others. The nursing staff, comprised, on average, one trained sister and one staff nurse on each ward. The remaining nursing staff were mostly from St. John's or the Red Cross Ambulance Services and many were directed to work at the hospital during the war years. Some well known local nurses were:

Janet Waugh	Diana Darling	Doreen Leader
Vivian Jarvis	Natalie Barling	Mary Taylor
Mary Lomas and her sister	Heather Tyler	Ruth Hobbs and her sister

Civilian admissions were restricted to air raid casualties, tuberculosis and maternity patients and treatment of epidemic outbreaks in evacuee homes of the elderly. Some payment was required for their stay in hospital.

The laundry ran into grave difficulties. Originally fitted out in 1921 to cope with 200 patients and 25 staff it was now washing over 6,000 articles a week. Miss B. Swann was the poor Laundry Superintendent and her life must have been hell!

The new boiler house in "C" Block, fitted with four White Rose low pressure boilers, and the new mortuary, were opened in April, 1942. The old post mortem slab was sent to Bury St. Edmunds Public Assistance Institute and the old mortuary building in "A" Block was used as a provisions store: I wonder how many people knew that at the time?

"C" Block kitchen was opened in March and provided all the patients' food. "A" Block kitchen remained open and provided food for the staff dining room. Electric food trolleys were supplied for "B" and "C" Block wards.

The old disinfector was working overtime removing the local troops of their unwanted guests for which a charge of 10s. 6d. per load was made.

The pig sty must have been empty for the kitchen swill was sold for 6d for a five gallon drum.

Dr. Platts was appointed house officer in April. She married Dr. Arden Jones a year later. They are both very well known for their excellent work over so many years.

On 1st May a light trailer fire pump was obtained and the staff trained in its use. This was great fun and it was surprising the muddles they got into. They did put some fires out and got many wet shirts doing so.

Mrs. Benson and her staff opened the Red Cross Library which was appreciated so very much by the patients and staff and their good work continued for some years after the war.

During the summer a Staff Entertainments Committee was formed and regular concerts were given for the patients. The hospital staff concert party gave a public performance in the Turner Hall on 22nd November, 1943, and these annual concerts continue until the present day. E.N.S.A. also started giving concerts in May, 1942, and these continued at intervals for two or three years after the war ended. Lavine, a ventriloquist, was often at the hospital. He became a big name in the entertainment world after the war ended and television took a hold of our lives.

In June the Pathology Laboratory was recognised as an area laboratory providing services for the County and County Institutions. The X-ray Department also provided a service for patients from the Isle of Ely area and for this service a charge of £1. 1s. 0d. per X-ray was made.

Ward A2 was used as a Sick Staff and Officers Ward (upstairs and Maternity and Labour Ward downstairs). On 4th July, small boys stole money and items from the Church: I bet the Rev. Gardener said a prayer for them!

The pack store, for service patients' clothing and personal effects, was brought into use on 14th August and a Military Registrar's Office consisting of one sergeant and one private was opened about the same time.

St. Phillip's Hall was used as a recreation room for service patients and a large local house "Heathside" was opened for rehabilitation patients in October.

It is interesting to note that it was agreed at this time that if life was prejudiced by the thirteen mile journey to Cambridge or Bury St. Edmunds, accident cases could be taken to either the White Lodge EMS or the Rous Memorial Hospital in Newmarket. The only difference today is that we do not even have the Rous Memorial Hospital.

It was reported that there was a lack of cigarettes and chocolate in the NAAFI and that a Military Police force consisting of two NCOs and four ORs would be attached to the hospital: maybe the two things were connected in some way. Orderlies were men from the Pioneer Corps and from the French Ambulance Unit, who had been working in the fighting lines and had come back to this country for a much needed rest.

At the end of the statistical year 31st December, 1942, there were 551 patients in the hospital. The total admissions for the past year was 5,289 and of these 4,658 had been service patients.

```
       Norwich cases: 91 casualties      93
                      sick              317
                                        410
```

Beds occupied (including 50 cases of tuberculosis)   551

The costing statement for the year at the end of the financial year to 31st March, 1943 was:

```
       Overhead charges           £55,692.
       Maintenance                £28,996.
                          Total   £84,688
```

The average bed complement 714   (considerably increased by the
The average bed occupancy   507   use of emergency beds)

"Heathfields", another large house in Bury Road, Newmarket, was requisitioned for the duration of the war and, in September, 1942, opened for the rehabilitation of patients.

In March, 1942, a ward-type block, purpose-built as nurses' accommodation, was opened in "C" Block and the nurses from Cleveland House moved into it. This was a big improvement. By April, 1943, both "Heathfields" and "Cleveland" were being used for the rehabilitation of military patients. The use of these houses was flexible and, by November, 1943, "Cleveland" house was again being used for nurses' accommodation.

At this point I think we should pause and reflect on what had been accomplished since the first items of equipment started to arrive late in 1939.

In about two years a completely new Emergency Hospital had been built, staffed and equipped, with a bed complement in excess of 700 beds. While the extensive building work was in progress, patients were being admitted and treated in increasing numbers in the old "A" Block accommodation. This was truly a remarkable feat, in so short a time, and my admiration goes out, not only to the hospital staff, who must have improvised in an amazing way, but also to the voluntary services, the builders and so many local people who were involved and without whose help the project could not have been achieved.

Dedication to duty must have been extraordinary and a wonderful "esprit de corps" existed. I am told despite the gloom of war a very happy atmosphere prevailed which is so essential for a successful hospital. Newmarket General Hospital has always been known as a very happy hospital and is so today and I am sure the root cause goes back to those day of 1942 and the so many wonderful staff who have worked in it.

By the end of 1942 the pattern of the hospital had been settled and from 1943 onwards, until the creation of the National Health Service in 1948, there was a pattern of consolidation and general improvement to existing services.

Towards the end of 1942 application had been made to the General Nursing Council to open a Nursing Training School. Following the usual visit and inspection of the hospital facilities, the application was refused.

Rationing was strict and food in short supply. A large number of chickens were kept on spare ground near "B" Block and supplied eggs and food for the patients. Although we ate much less food then a system of barter grew up. We were working hard and it is considered that the nation was a lot healthier than it is today. For example, the incidence of heart disease has greatly increased since those days.

1943 *New Services*

In April the hospital staff organised a collection for "Wings for Victory" and although the target was set at £500 they raised £1,706. 3s. 6d. which was considered a very large amount at the time.

A dental surgery was opened in the spring of 1943 and there was a general build up of tuberculosis cases,

A new boiler had to be fitted in Cleveland House and the Newmarket Lawn Tennis Club offered membership to the doctors and nurses at a fee of £3. 3s. 0d. per season.

Mr. Rowlands was sent for duty at Tilbury docks for one week. Miss E. M. Goodchild and Mr. J. S. Garmory were appointed clerks and on 28th August Mr. E. S. Jamieson took over the Fracture Centre from Mr. J. Grant Bonnin. The hospital was reported quiet at this time. Mr. E. S. Jamieson and Miss M. Welply will always be remembered for their many years of excellent service in the orthopaedic, poliomyelitis, physiotherapy and casualty departments.

Under the original guidance of Miss Hayter and, later, Miss S. M. Stevens, the physiotherapy department built up a fine reputation for their work and as early as June 1943 the department was chosen to give short courses, twice a year, for masseurs in patient's rehabilitation.

On 13th July the remainder of Major Beaty's paddock was requisitioned by the Ministry of Health for the rehabilitation of military patients and he did not like this at all. The paddock was not handed over to the hospital until 8th June, 1944. It was not nice that at about 10 p.m. on the night of the handover five or six of Major Beaty's cattle, including two bullocks, escaped into the hospital grounds. They made a great mess and there were few people who thought it was an accident. Messrs. Hollands built a long and high brick boundary wall after this!

Local people reserved accommodation in their homes for the use of relatives visiting patients in the hospital. A register was kept for a number of years and this kindness was very greatly appreciated by the relatives.

At last during the summer of 1943, the old laundry was given some help. New equipment to the value of £2,250 was installed and since this required a better steam supply a separate Cochrane boiler and boiler house was built alongside the laundry building. This worked at 100lbs pressure whereas the Lancashire boiler only provided at 60lbs

The increase in the number of tuberculosis patients continued and by November Ward B4 and B6 had been set aside for this specialty. Then, fresh air was one form of treatment and open verandas were built in Wards B2, B4 and B6 and about six outside small chalets were obtained. The patients lived in this outside accommodation. On 13th October, 1944, the Ministry of Health made White Lodge EMS a receiving centre for tuberculosis patients from the other hospitals in the area.

Towards the end of 1943 civilian ear, nose and throat patients (ENT) were being admitted under Mr. R. Williamson, for which a charge of £2. 2s. 0d. per case was made.

A number of Italian prisoners of war had arrived. Some of these were skilled tradesmen and did very good work for the hospital.

1944 A Busier Year

In 1944 the hospital became very much busier. Troops were returning from the Far East and a large number of malaria cases were being admitted. There was a general increase in the number of outpatients and in the work of the medical, surgical, E.N.T. and fracture departments. Extra beds were put up in the wards and a number of cases had to be diverted to Black Notley Hospital in Colchester. The bed state of available beds was:

Bed complement including 48 T.B. and 4 Maternity beds	669
By crowding in extra beds	71
Beds in Physiotherapy Department in emergency	26
Beds in Occupational Therapy in emergency	_26_
Total	792

In March a convoy of 79 overseas cases were admitted and malaria cases were still being received.

In June the Air Ministry relinquished Oakfield House and application was made for it to be used as a nurses' home. This was refused.

On 11th August twenty-one children suffering from gastroenteritis were admitted from a childrens' hostel in Walsham-le-Willows - they were very ill - five died before admission and two whilst in hospital and local people were scared by the press reports and rumour. Penicillin had just been made available and its use was restricted to service patients. A little over-ordering enabled the physician in charge to save some of the children's lives. Penicillin and intravenous feeding made a breakthrough in treating such epidemics.

Major Bailey Hawkins took over the duties of local transport officer and Mr. J. Wheeler resigned from the House Committee.

Providing meals for staff on night duty has always been a problem in hospitals. This was always done by the cooks in the catering department forming a rota for night duty but the arrangement caused difficulties during holidays and when staff were short. In October the catering staff refused to form the rota and efforts were made to recruit competent part-time night cooks. This was not always possible and the difficulty remained until some years later when a microwave vending machine was installed.

On 1st November five more children were admitted from The Grove Home in Walsham-le-Willows and during the month convoys of casualties started to arrive from overseas. Between the 11th and 13th November 186 wounded German soldiers were admitted and an air convoy of 81 cases of British and Allied casualties arrived from Newmarket Heath. The operating theatres were working twelve hours a day for a fortnight and there were 711 patients in the hospital.

1945 *Peace comes to Europe*

In February, 1945, 109 German prisoners of war remained in the hospital: they occupied three wards. Osborne House, Newmarket was taken over as a nurses' hostel on 15th February and it was so occupied until 19th November.

On 27th February Mr. Bertie Newton, who was well known locally and was a member of the Hospital Committee for many years, suffered a heart attack whilst attending a meeting in the Board Room, and died. He was succeeded by Captain H. R. King, CBE, JP.

On 24th February a convoy of 145 prisoner of war stretcher cases arrived at the hospital. It was reported that 213 German P.O.W. patients still remained and although staff were still directed to the hospital there was a general shortage at this time.

The danger and difficulties of moving stretcher cases up the wooden stairs to Ward A2 was reported and it was recommended that a lift should be provided as a matter of urgency.

Major Bailey Hawkins reported to the March meeting of the Hospital Committee on the work of the Civil Defence Vehicles up to 31st March, 1945 :

Number of convalescent cases and casualties conveyed   7,219
Mileage   43,843
Petrol used   3,655¼ gals.

The convoys continued to arrive and on 2nd May 100 military cases were admitted to the hospital and a further 119 on 17th May.

Hostilities ceased in Europe on 8th May, 1945, and although the war in the Far East continued for a further year the whole nature of the hospital slowly changed. The spirit of freedom was high in both patients and staff: it was great to be alive. The boys were returning with small gratuities and everyone wanted to go home. Beer of a sort was plentiful and there was a shortage of pianos in the pubs. The students gradually returned to the University and brought a great spirit of fun to Cambridge. The "Cherry Tree", which had always been run so well by the Coleman family, became a sort of annex to the hospital and both staff and patients spent many happy times there.

The work in the hospital continued and on 23rd May Mr. J. Rowlands was called up to the Army. When he first came to the hospital there was no surgical instruments and equipment for him to use. He had been in private practice and loaned a large amount of his personal equipment to the hospital. This had not been replaced and he threatened to take it all with him. I think his call up was cancelled but it was quite a long time before he was compensated for his equipment.

The improvements in the laundry were completed in May and the post of Head Laundress advertised. Alas, the poor old steam engine had been worked to death and in November it had to be completely overhauled by Messrs. Webbs of Exning. In June the space at the back of the laundry was covered in to form a shelter for the patients in "C" Block.

The A.R.P. and contamination centre, which were the original casual wards, were handed back to the hospital by the Civil Defence on 24th May, 1945. The first aid post was handed back by the Red Cross on 1st March, 1946.

Over 100 service patients had been transferred to other hospitals all over the County: this was done so that they would be near their homes. There were 461 patients in the hospital at this time but in July a convoy of 119 cases arrived from overseas and the numbers increased to 551. Valuable assistance was given by the voluntary personnel, trained under the various Civil Defence services.

The first hospital Open Day was held on 1st July. All the wards were opened to the public as well as theatres, x-ray, physiotherapy and pathology. A few of the staff present on the day were Colonel Watson, Dr. Hawes and Miss Welply, Mr. Jamieson, Mr. Thompson (Pharmacy) and Mr. Williamson. This became an annual event.

Towards the end of July the hospital became much quieter. The number of patients had reduced to 450 and these were mostly long stay cases. On 19th July the shortage of nursing staff was being felt and Ward B2 was closed. This was the real start of a general shortage of nursing and technical staff which was to become acute in many hospitals all over the country. The direction of staff to hospitals had ceased and staff had to be recruited locally.

The Army had provided the ambulance service throughout the War and as they closed down and more civilian patients were admitted to the hospital they left a real problem. In June a few very old converted ambulances and cars were obtained from the Civil Defence and Mr. A. Humphries, who had been the chimney sweep, was engaged as a driver. Parkers Garage in Field Terrace Road was purchased by the hospital to house the vehicles and Jim Milward's garage, somehow, kept them on the road. In September the American ambulance service based at Cambridge, who had been doing all the long distance work, notified that they were closing down. The existing old vehicles were not suitable for this work and an urgent recommendation for more comfortable ambulances was made. This was refused by the Ministry of Health and this difficulty remained for a long time.

In the autumn of 1945 the War Office was asked for permission to remove the air raid shelters between the wards so that the appearance of the grounds could be improved. This was refused and the shelters were only removed when they fell to pieces, through neglect, some few years later.

In October 143 orthopaedic and peripheral nerve injury cases were transferred from Leys School, Cambridge. The centre was closed down and the orthopaedic cases sent to Mr. Jamieson's department. Mr. Butler was in charge of the male nerve injury cases: some nursing staff were transferred to White Lodge EMS with the patients.

The first mention of Trade Unions in Newmarket Hospital was in October 1945 when the National Federation of Building Trade Operators negotiated for better pay for porters.

By the autumn White Lodge EMS was working closely with Addenbrooke's Hospital in Cambridge and a strong move was made to make it an annex of that hospital. At a meeting held on 25th September the Ministry of Health did not agree and made it quite clear that White Lodge should work independently of Addenbrooke's. Despite rumours of closure it remains open and independent today.

In November the Dean X-ray unit was replaced by a Westinghouse 500 M.A. fixed unit (ex-lease lend). Mr. Bill Knappet purchased the old Dean set as scrap.

About this time the general practitioners were notified that the hospital was open for the regular admission of certain classes of civilian patients.

A small convoy of sixteen service cases arrived at the end of November and an appreciable number of repatriated prisoners of war from Japan were being admitted.

1946 *Shortages of Staff*

By the end of January, 1946, a large number of the nursing staff had applied for release. These were members of the Civil Nursing Reserve and the rule was for those with more than three years' service, they could go at once. For those with more than two years' service, they could go after the end of April. It was not possible for the work of the hospital to carry on without restricting admissions. The nursing staff continued to resign and it was necessary to close Ward B3 (gastric) and Ward C6 (fracture) on 25th February. The patients were distributed amongst other wards. At this time the shortage of nursing staff was a national problem and whilst recruitment was easier for the central hospitals in the cities, those in rural areas had difficulty in keeping going and as time went by had to resort to all sorts of recruitment schemes. The shortages went on for a long time.

On 28th February Oakfield House was handed back to the owners, the Calcutta Club, and the cost of dilapidation paid. A wooden sectional hut which had been assembled in the grounds was transferred to the hospital.

A nursery for children under two years old was opened in the tin roof building at the end of A3 ward for the West Suffolk County Council and sixteen children transferred from Walnut Tree Hospital in Sudbury. A sandpit was built for the children near the old mortuary.

Minutes of meetings of that time show that in April staff recruitment difficulties were growing. No applications were received from an advertisement in the "Daily Telegraph" for a Food Supervisor. Corporal E. Carter wrote asking what salary he would receive when he returned to work at the hospital from the forces. It was not possible to give him an answer. At the meeting held on 26th April it was recorded:

> "all domestics at White Lodge Emergency Hospital receive wages at the rate of 1s. 4d. per hour for normal time and 1s. 6d. per hour overtime rate. (Before 8 a.m. and after 5 p.m. and for Sunday work)."

The Ministry of Health granted the continued use of Wards B4 and B6 and the chalets for tuberculosis cases, under the care of Consultant Physician Dr. Arden Jones, and sanctioned the admission of E.N.T. cases from Addenbrooke's Hospital. Heathfield House and Cleveland House were de-requisitioned and handed back to the owners in May.

Victory celebrations were held on 8th June, 1946. During the month of May the Army P.T. Instructor was recalled and Mr. V. R. Parkinson recruited in his place. Ward B5 was closed because of staff shortage. The transfer of female orthopaedic and peripheral nerve injury cases from Addenbrooke's Hospital ceased.

Some of the members of the Hospital Committee were then Mr. J. B. Coster, Mr. H.R. Buck, Mr. J. G . Taylor and Mrs. F. Ramsay. The Committee's attention was drawn to the poor condition of the wards which had received little attention during the war years. To make life even more difficult the District Auditor's reports were now being received.

Miss Lithgow resigned her post as Matron to take effect in September. She was succeeded by Miss R. E. Finch and Miss Sarbutt was appointed first Assistant Matron.

By 18th July the number of patients had fallen to 286. The nursing staff available was only 88 and Wards C7 (male surgical), B1 (male medical) and A1 (ENT) had to be closed. Because of the lack of midwives there was a real danger of a breakdown in maternity bookings.

Resident domestic staff were living in a ward divided by cubicle curtains to make a sort of private room. The conditions were bad and staff became in short supply.

On 18th July the General Nursing Council gave provisional approval for White Lodge Emergency Hospital to be a Training School of Student Nurses. This was most necessary and there was much work to do for the first intake of student nurses in the summer of 1948.

It was reported that six inches of rain fell during a storm on 25th August and most of the wards were flooded.

Addenbrooke's Hospital was also experiencing difficulties and in September arrangements were made for some of their surgical and ENT cases, on their waiting lists, living in the Newmarket area, to be admitted to White Lodge Emergency Hospital. Ward C5 (male orthopaedic) was closed.

On 8th November the use of St. Fabians' estate was obtained as a Nurses' Home. The owner, Mr. P. Hammond, who also owned the present Barclay's Bank premises and of Hammond Bank, died and the Hospital Authority negotiated the purchase of the estate.

One race night in October, 1946, a gentleman, who had been racing and was rather under the weather, wandered into the hospital grounds. He opened the door and saw a number of articles of personal clothing from which he stole all the valuables and went on his way. Unbeknown to him he had walked into the theatre surgeons' changing room and had stolen all the money, a gold watch and other articles from Mr. Rowlands' and other staffs' pockets. Mr. Rowlands was operating at the time and when he finished he was most unhappy to find all his valuables missing. He immediately locked all the theatre doors and called the police. Only two members of the staff had gone home. They were recalled and questioned at length by the police, since they and Mr. Rowlands were convinced that a member of the theatre staff on duty at the time was the thief. The staff were given a bad time. Some weeks later a thief was arrested in London and was found to possess Mr. Rowlands' watch. He admitted being in Newmarket and stealing the property but he refused to believe he had robbed a surgeon during the course of an operation. He was very upset!

There must have been many funny incidents over the years and long may they continue. On another race night a well-oiled racegoer wandered into the hospital grounds looking for accommodation for the night. He got hopelessly lost, which was easy to do, and eventually looked through the french window of one of the wards. He saw a very comfortable bed so he opened the door, undressed and enjoyed a good night's sleep. In the morning he was given breakfast, shown the ablutions and it was most unfortunate that I was talking to the sister in charge of the ward, in her office, when the gentleman knocked on her office door and asked her how much he owed for the night's stay? Now some ward sisters are known to be dragons, but I have never seen one take off with so much bad language and threats against the poor man. She knew she would never live it down and I am afraid I made sure she didn't!

By October the nature of the hospital had started to change. The numbers of emergency service patients were decreasing and being replaced by much older civilian patients. A hospital for German P.O.W. was opened in Diss in Norfolk and by June, 1947, all service patients had been withdrawn from the hospital.

The shortage of nursing staff continued and as an aid to recruitment hospital transport was made available during the evenings to take the nurses to and from Cambridge for an evening out. This continued for two or three years.

The whole of ward A1 was converted into a maternity block and opened on 6th December. It was reported at the time that the furniture was in a very poor condition. Ward C1 was converted to an outpatient department which was a much needed improvement.

The condition of the makeshift ambulances and cars continued to give trouble. The local Red Cross agreed to loan an ambulance on Thursdays which was the busy tuberculosis outpatient day. They were paid 3d. per mile for the service which continued for a long time. Public transport was in short supply and patients had to be collected from the villages and taken home at the end of the clinic. The ambulances made a circular tour of the villages to pick up patients and take them home afterwards.

1947 Back to Normal

A 16 mm film projector was purchased in January, 1947, films were hired and the engineer and another member of staff toured the wards giving film shows to the patients.

By 23rd May the number of patients in the hospital had fallen to 202.

During the early months of 1947 all the military staff were withdrawn and their duties transferred to the hospital Clerk and Steward. Colonel Watson retired on 18th March and Dr. Hawes acted as Medical Superintendent until Air Vice Marshal Kelly was appointed on 29th August.

There had been so many changes and new senior staff appointed that it was not surprising there was a general upheaval of the administrative control of the Hospital. This was eventually sorted out: medical matters by the Medical Superintendent, nursing matters by the Matron and administration by the Clerk and Steward.

In August the Ministry of Health requested a unit be opened for the late treatment of poliomyelitis cases. Ward C3 (male) and ward C7 (female) were used for this purpose. The unit was put under the control of Mr. E. S. Jamieson, the senior Orthopaedic Surgeon. Six iron lungs were delivered and the staff trained in their use. A mobile team of two nurses, trained in the use of the iron lung, were available with this equipment to go to the aid of polio cases, in emergency, anywhere in East Anglia. They were sent out on four occasions. When the polio unit opened twenty-three cases were admitted from all over East Anglia and this increased the bed state, which in August, was 242. Six very long wicker carriages were received in which polio cases could be taken round the hospital grounds during the summer months.

The iron lungs were made in America and could be operated manually in case of an electric mains failure. Mr. K. A. G. Allison, the Hospital Engineer, trained the staff in the manual use. He had difficulty in obtaining spare parts which had to be obtained from America. He told me they found an important electrical relay had been made by Magnetic Devices Ltd. who were only a matter of yards from the hospital: there was no difficulty in obtaining future spares. It is interesting that some of those iron lungs have been found, modified, and put back into use in the hospital Chest Unit of today.

Little mention has been made of the considerable help the hospital has always received from the local people and voluntary organisations and of the numerous gifts which have been and continue to be received. They have given great encouragement to the hospital staff and helped to create the happy atmosphere for which the hospital has always been well known.

Since the beginning of September, 1939, over 30,000 patients had been admitted to the hospital and the numerous letters of thanks and appreciation was evidence of the good work done.

At the end of 1946 Miss Finch, the new Matron, reported to the Committee on the very bad condition of the nurses' accommodation and the general shortage of nursing staff. The condition of the wards and furniture was very poor. The hospital was then in the period between the end of the war and the introduction of the National Health Service on 5th July, 1948. The whole question was under review - it was expensive and long term. The same difficulties were being experienced in most other hospitals: there was very little money available and, in my view, it would have been more difficult NOT to have introduced the National Health Service.

Chapter Eight

THE NATIONAL HEALTH SERVICE
SECONDARY CARE OR HOSPITAL SERVICES

Unfortunately, the records of the hospital for the first few years of the National Health Service, introduced by the National Health Service Act, 1946, have not been traced and I have had to rely on memory to some extent.

In 1948 the East Anglian Regional Hospital Board (No. 4) was formed to administer the hospital services in East Anglia. Its area consisted of the Counties of Norfolk, Suffolk and Cambridgeshire and the headquarters were based in Cambridge. Dr. I. B. Ewan was appointed Regional Medical Officer and the names of some old friends in his department included Dr. Todd White, who I believe married a Nurse Pearmain who was working at White Lodge Hospital, Mr. Vic Minter and Geoff Hurst, all very good administrators.

The Region was divided into fifteen to twenty Groups of Hospitals administered by Hospital Management Committees (HMC). The South West (No. 1) Group HMC was based at White Lodge Hospital and occupied the present administrative and telephone exchange premises in "A" Block. The Group headquarters contained the following departments:

Chairman	Captain H. R. King, CBE, JP.
Group Secretary	Brigadier T. R. Henry.
Group Treasurer	Mr. G. Meadowcroft.
Group Engineer	Mr. H. Merrin (based at Fulbourn Hospital)
Group Supplies Officer	Mr. N. E. Kendall (based in Ward B5).

Other Group departments, such as Group Catering, Group Fire and Group Building Supervision were added as time went by.

Mr. N. E. Kendall had worked at the Public Assistance Institution for a number of years as Assistant Master to Mr. E. S. Heasman, who was Master for many years and was now the Hospital Clerk and Steward. It was nice to have him back.

The administrative work which was carried out by the West Suffolk County Council during the war years was transferred to the new Group headquarters and their responsibilities for hospitals ceased. They continued to administer the primary care services, viz ambulance service, health centres, maternity and child welfare and home nursing, etc.

The name of the hospital was changed to Newmarket General Hospital in 1951.

The original No. 1 Group was very large and as elsewhere contained the mental health service hospitals. This was effected in an attempt to break down the isolation in which the mental health service had tended to function. The original Group contained the following hospitals:

> Paxton Park Maternity Hospital, St. Neots.
> Fulbourn Psychiatric Hospital.
> Riversfield SubNormal Hospital, St. Neots.
> Little Plumstead Hospital.
> Tower Hospital, Ely.
> Grange Maternity Hospital, Ely.
> Huntingdon County Hospital.
> Cardigan Street Nursing Home.
> Primrose Lane Maternity Hospital, Huntingdon.
> Walnut Tree Hospital.
> Cambridge Chest Clinic.
> Saffron Walden General Hospital.
> St. James' Hospital, Saffron Walden.
> Royston General Hospital.
> Royston Maternity Hospital
> Newmarket General Hospital.
> Exning Isolation Hospital.

The Group departments to administer these hospitals were very small. For example, the officers in the Group Secretary's Department were:

> Brigadier T. R. Henry   Group Secretary,
> Mr. G. S. Pearmain   Deputy Group Secretary,
> Miss Challice   Secretary,
> Miss Nash   Typist.

Fulbourn Hospital alone contained almost 1,000 beds and it soon became clear that the Group was far too large for proper administration. The specialized mental and subnormal hospitals were withdrawn in 1949 and formed another separate Group (No. 13) based at Fulbourn Hospital. Mr. C. Mitchell, who had been the well-established Hospital Clerk and Steward, became the No. 13 Group Secretary. The Group officers had been appointed for all the hospitals and apart from the Group Secretary they continued to be responsible for them. They held joint appointments for both of the Groups. For convenience sake both Groups were called South West No. 1 and 13 Group Hospital Management Committee. They worked quite separately.

No. 1 Group being based at Newmarket General Hospital caused difficulties for the staff working at the patient level since the Group officers became involved with the day to day work. However, their interest did release funds and allow the hospital to develop which was so necessary at that time.

In order to involve the Group Secretary in the day to day work of the hospitals it was decided to make him hold the joint appointment of Group Secretary and Hospital Secretary of the main hospital to which the Group headquarters was attached. This caused unrest and friction since the Clerk and Steward was the Hospital Secretary under a different name. This was a bad arrangement and caused many difficulties and, in my opinion, should not have been implemented until those in post retired or moved on: even then it was a bad arrangement and was rescinded when the first reorganisation came in 1974.

Mr. E. S. Heasman was the Clerk and Steward at Newmarket General Hospital and had been so for a very long time. Difficulties with the Group Secretary continued until Mr. Heasman retired on 31st March, 1951. His duties were then taken over by the Group Secretary, Brigadier T. R. Henry.

At the end of the war Newmarket General Hospital, like so many other hospitals, was run down and badly needed renovating and updating to a general hospital. There was a general shortage of equipment and the introduction of the National Health Service provided the necessary funds for by 1960 the expenditure on the health service was at a level thirty per cent greater than in 1949.

1954 *Nurse Staffing Problems*

By November, 1954, the General Nurses' Training School had been transferred to St. Fabians. The first Sister Tutor was a Miss E.M. Spiller. She was followed by Miss Butler, who used to ride a horse around St. Fabians' grounds in her spare time. She fell off one day and hurt her head and left the hospital shortly afterwards. She was replaced by Miss Meredith.

The first Nurses' Prizegiving had been held in 1952 when Professor Maxwell had presented the prizes and certificates.

The recruitment of nurses for the Training School was very difficult and a number of determined recruitment drives were made in the areas of Newmarket, Haverhill, Soham and also in the Newmarket side of Cambridge. These drives consisted of nursing talks and displays in prominent shop windows and leaflets through householder letter boxes. Recruitment advertisements were put on all the local cinema screens and in the newspapers. Permission was obtained from the Regional Hospital Board to advertise on Anglia Television. Mr. Leo Maycock, a member of the theatre staff, took photographs of the theatre and other departments of the hospital and slides were made up. Advertising on Anglia television was expensive but did result in over thirty potential recruits. Eventually the Ministry of Health forbade all such advertising and so Newmarket General Hospital was about the first and last hospital to do this.

The British Red Cross Society and other voluntary organisations were a great help in these recruitment drives and I remember putting an iron lung on display at the Rutland Hill, Newmarket, one Saturday. Miss Vivien Jarvis and hospital staff gave demonstrations in its use. Much interest was shown by the people of the town.

In April the hospital fire arrangements were reviewed in conjunction with the County and Newmarket Fire Brigade chiefs. A new fire alarm system and appliances were recommended and Mr. Deasley, a hospital painter, engaged to maintain and service the fire extinguishers and equipment. Regular fire lectures and practices were arranged and a very good relationship built up between the hospital staff and the local fire brigade.

By September the new 100 line telephone exchange had been installed and was a very necessary improvement. The telephonists who gave excellent service and performed many additional duties were, during the daytime, Miss D. Freeman and Miss D. Mowl and, at night, Mr. Fred Milne and Mr. Ronald. Mrs. I. Darval was the relief operator. When not operating the telephone exchange she worked in the medical records department.

The Almoner was given a Samaritan Fund from which she could make immediate payments for travelling expenses, etc. to patients and visitors.

As the number of patients passing through the hospital increased so did the number of patients' records. Storage space was scarce and the hospital Medical Staff Committee could not agree on the length of time these records should be kept. The result was that they were stored in odd corners and in the old air raid shelters all over the hospital, which was not good for the records or for the staff who had to handle them. The problem remained for many years and may well do so today.

In April, 1954, the Group Secretary, Brigadier T. R. Henry, retired and was succeeded by Mr. A. W. Youngs.

In the same month, Miss M. Welply was taken ill and remained so for some time. This created difficulties in staffing the Casualty Department and it had to be closed from time to time. Mr. E. S. Jamieson and Miss M. Welply had run the casualty service singlehanded since its existence and the hospital owes much to their loyal service. Miss Welply did not completely recover and she resigned in January, 1964. She was very much missed.

In May the first "Cross Infection Committee" was set up and the Nurses' Training School badge was adopted as the Hospital Badge. This month also saw the letting of the first contract to service the specialized equipment in the Physiotherapy Department. The contractors were Messrs. General Radiological Ltd. at the agreed price of £5. per quarter. The work in the Hospital Engineer's department had increased and although they did the day to day maintenance in the department a more specialised service was required.

The numbers of patients in the TB wards were increasing and the Red Cross hut in "B" Block was used as a recreation room. Mrs. O'Callaghan from Burwell and the Red Cross workers furnished and maintained the hut.

During the spring of 1954 television sets started to arrive for the wards - the cost was met from the Hospital Free Monies with help from the Newmarket Journal Xmas Fund and other voluntary services. The programme took quite some time to complete and was very much appreciated by the patients. TV sets were hired from Radio Rentals for some of the wards.

In May the Hospital held another Open Day, with the Newmarket Town Band in attendance. Although the emphasis of recruitment was on nursing staff there was a general shortage in all departments. Wards had to be closed and junior medical staff were particularly difficult to recruit.

Despite these shortages at this time a wonderful spirit existed amongst the staff of the hospital. The relief after the war years was still being felt and the staff worked long hours with little reward. This was particularly so in the Nursing Recruitment Drives but we all had a great deal of fun.

There was some dissatisfaction amongst the nursing staff about the lack of entertainment in the town when off duty and from 21st July a staff bus service to and from Cambridge was introduced.

In July Mr. R. Williamson, Consultant ENT Surgeon, was Chairman of the House Committee and the elaborate Chairman's Chair, a relic from the Board of Guardians, had the letters N.B.G. (Newmarket Board of Guardians) engraved on the back, above the Chairman's head. One day a very annoyed member of the Committee shouted at the chairman that the letters were most appropriate for him. The letters were quickly removed by the carpenter the following morning!

In September provisions were still controlled and the junior medical staff requested an extra sugar ration for their quarters. A supplementary allowance of 3lbs. 11oz. a week was made to cover occasional meals for non-residents and night work.

At this time, where possible, all inventory items were marked and inventories checked at regular intervals. An engraving machine was purchased for marking cutlery, etc. Crockery was marked by a special paint and all linen marked in the hospital sewing room. It's a shame something like this is not done today: the cost of inventory deficiencies at 31st March, 1954, was £105. 6s. 10d.

The Bishop of St. Edmundsbury & Ipswich presented the prizes at the Nurses' Prizegiving and afterwards spoke to patients from the Church via a new extension of the patients' pillow radio system. From then on the Church Services were broadcast to the patients on Sunday mornings.

In September the Maternity Unit in Ward A1 was renovated. The unit was moved to temporary accommodation in Ward C7 while the work was in progress. The staff worked under considerable difficulties.

In this same month the Hospital Cricket team won the "Pudney Cup". In fact they won it twice. The cup was given by Mr. Pudney, Chairman of the Newmarket Urban District Council, and the knockout cricket competition amongst local firms and organisations was arranged by Council staff who laid a concrete wicket on the Severals for the purpose. A lot of teams from business and other organisations entered and quite large crowds of people watched the matches during the summer evenings. It is a shame that Severals is not used in a similar way today. Some members of the hospital team were Dr. Blackiston, Consultant Anaesthetist, Mr. G. Meadowcroft, Taffy Hughes from

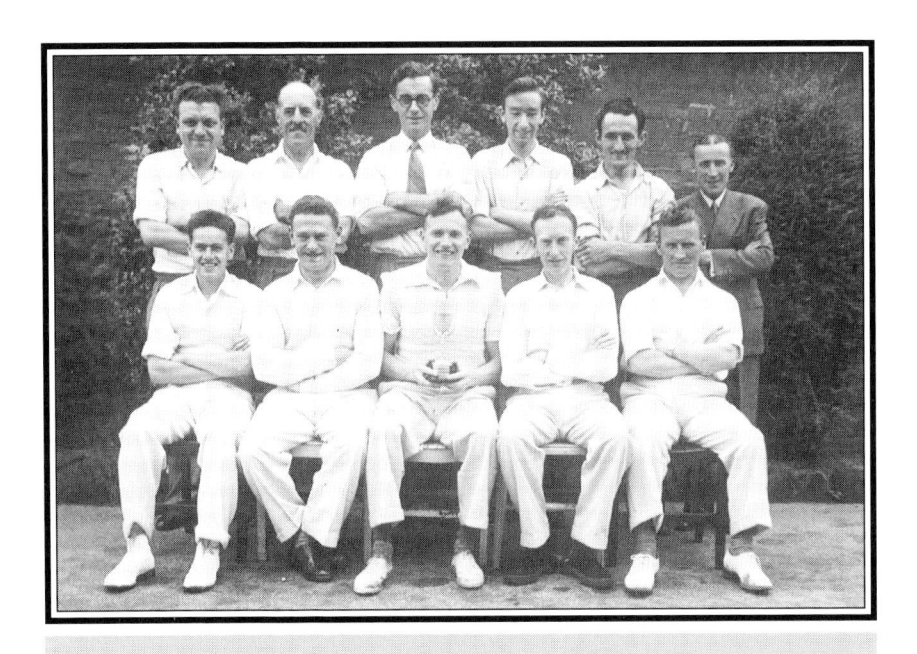

**The Pudney Cup Winning Team
1954**

the Treasurer's Department, Mr. W. Hobbs, the Hospital Pharmacist and myself. Mr. K.A.G. Allison, the Hospital Engineer, insists to this day that he alone won the cup. The fact was that someone dropped out of the team at the last minute and he was put in to make the number up. He fielded at long stop and only saw the ball once when he bent down to stop it and it went through his legs for four runs. He still says he hit the winning hit. I know that the bowler accidentally hit Mr. Allison's bat and the ball flew off to the boundary. He was looking in the opposite direction at the time and it became known that that was the first and last time he ever played cricket. It was great fun at the time.

In October Dr. Gregg was the Consultant Radiologist and he requested an extension be made to the X-ray Department by taking in a small portion of the theatre building. The department was very cramped and as the work increased this was a very necessary extension.

The laundry services in the No. 1 Group were presenting difficulties and in November it was agreed the service should be centralised at Newmarket at a cost of £4,750. This would include a large, new central linen store, new washing machines, tumble dryers, rapid twin press and a gap in the existing calender. Mrs. Curtis was the Laundry Superintendent at the time and Mr. Rolfe and Mr. Barnard-Smith did the work in the soiled linen and wash room. A lorry driven by Mr. Tomlin from Fulbourn Hospital was used to take the large baskets to and from the other hospitals in the Group and this arrangement continued quite well for a number of years.

Mrs. E. Mason was the Kitchen Superintendent for a long time. Shortly after 1948 the Regional Hospital Board appointed Messrs. J. Lyons as Consultant Catering Advisor. Their hospital representative was Mr. Turner who was very helpful. Complaints were being received about the standard of catering and the RHB accepted his recommendation that the main kitchen in "C" Block should be completely upgraded during 1954/55. Apart from new equipment and a change of use of some of the ancillary rooms a new quarry tile floor was laid throughout and also green ceramic wall tiles laid part way up the walls. The red floor tiles were laid first and were a wonderful improvement both for hygiene and for the appearance of the kitchen. There was an area of about 450 square yards of flooring and one Sunday morning, when the kitchen staff should have been at peace with the world, the new tiles in the main kitchen came up in a huge bubble to a height of about five feet and then burst in a shower of debris. Nobody had experienced anything like this before and there was a frightening noise and terrible mess everywhere. Unfortunately the news leaked to the national press and life was made hell for a time. As the work progressed it was decided, if possible, that the green wall tiles would be extended from floor to ceiling and this was done. Of course, the work exceeded the cash allowed by the RHB. Funds had been reserved to build a new Boiler House and maintenance workshop block in the future and it was decided to defer the maintenance block and use the cash to complete the wall tiling in the kitchen. It took about thirty years before the new workshop block was built and no marks can be given for this delay.

While the upgrading work was in progress the catering department was squeezed into the old kitchen in "A" Block and more use made of the ward kitchens which were really intended for beverages, light breakfasts and snacks. There were on average 200 patients and 175 resident staff in the hospital in December, 1954, and credit must be given not only to Mrs. Mason and her staff, but also to the nursing staff who helped so much in keeping the service going until the upgraded kitchen was available in "C" Block.

One calamity did occur. The new kitchen was not open for Christmas 1955 and it was not possible to cook about fifteen turkeys in the limited space in "A" Block kitchen. Mr. Trent, a local baker, offered to help and he cooked the turkeys and roast potatoes in his ovens at Wellington Street in the town. They were transported by van to the hospital and put into the heated food trollies with all the other trimmings. I was congratulating Mrs. Mason that the emergency system had worked when my telephone rang and a very irate Sister Cudden complained there was no Christmas turkey in the food trolley for the patients on her Ward C8. Panic reigned for a short time and I thought poor Mrs. Mason would have a heart attack. A telephone call to Mr. Trent left him in a black mood and upset because he assumed we accused him of pinching a turkey. The kitchen staff were questioned and were adamant that the turkey had been put into the food trolley. Sister Cudden insisted she had not got it and used rude words about the administrative and catering staff. In desperation I went to the ward with Mrs. Mason, opened the food trolley door and found the turkey on the bottom shelf! Mrs. Mason's face was full of relief and I was so sorry for her. Mr. Rowlands, Sister Cudden and her staff had indulged well but Christmas or not she had caused an unnecessary panic which did upset the catering staff and she was told so. Mr. Trent was very relieved that the missing turkey had been found but did not offer to help again.

I always thought Mrs. Mason and her team were the best Christmas dinner cooks in the District. Apart from the patients in the wards there were the resident staff dining rooms and the doctors', sisters' and nurses' quarters. Her staff included Mrs. Bartram (Head Cook), Mrs. D. Barton and I think Mr. Beeby had arrived by then. He is still at the hospital and is the best meat cook in the business.

"C" Block kitchen was opened early in 1955 and in order to improve the catering service a central dining room was opened in "C" Block for all the hospital staff. It was located close to the "C" Block kitchen, which allowed the Kitchen Superintendent and, shortly after, the Catering Officer to supervise the staff meals which had previously been provided in the Sisters' quarters and the Doctors' quarters in "A" Block and the non-resident staff and nurses' dining rooms in "C" Block. It also avoided hot meals being taken across the car parks and open grounds to the various dining rooms.

Mr. Turner, the Lyons Catering Advisor, recommended this scheme and it took many hours of negotiation with the medical and nursing staff before it was finally agreed that there should be one dining room only for all staff. I recall at the last moment Dr. Robertson, who was then the Chairman of the Medical Staff Committee, arrived at the office in quite a state. He said that the medical staff had not appreciated they would have to dine with the hospital staff generally and there had been an awful row. After another long discussion it was agreed that a screen should be provided at one end of the dining room so that the medical staff could discuss medical matters in private. A similar arrangement remains today.

The central dining was on the cafeteria basis, most of the food being provided from the main kitchen. It was opened in 1955 and was one of the very few of its kind in the country. It certainly was a first in East Anglia and many hospitals visited to see it in operation. I believe it is now an accepted method of staff catering and I find it interesting that, even today, many firms and organisations have not accepted the principle.

At this time the cost of feeding in all the other hospitals in the Group was being compared at regular intervals. It was £1. 7s. 6d. per head per week at Newmarket and this was considered high. The long term orthopaedic and TB patients were thought to be the reason for this. There had been a steady growth in the number of these patients.

The development and upgrading continued during 1955. Just before Christmas 1954 the Bury St. Edmunds Round Table made a gift of a 16mm film projector to the hospital. Films were hired and shown to the patients in the wards and to staff at regular intervals. The film shows were very much appreciated.

Mr. J. Rowlands, who had been the hospital Consultant Surgeon for the past fourteen years, resigned on 13th December, 1954. He was replaced by Mr. R. E. B. Tagart on 1st April, 1955. The hospital owes a great deal to both of these surgeons.

1955 *Comings and Goings*

Early in 1955 the Ministry of Health made a rule that staff working after retirement age should be subject to an annual review. Four members of the staff Mrs. Kerslake (Pharmacy), Mr. Copeman (Gardener), Mr. Rodman (Head Porter) and Mrs. Curtis (Laundry) were effected.

At the end of March the inventory checks showed losses to the value of £3. 3s. 3d. This was much better than the previous year and no doubt a few rockets had been delivered. In the same month the time clock was introduced to record the hours worked by ancillary staff. It was effective but caused a lot of work and was eventually abolished in favour of a better system.

On 22nd July Lord Derby presented the prizes at the Annual Nursing Prize Giving. In the same month the patients' call system was extended to all the wards. The Group Medical Advisory Committee was formed to coordinate the medical work in all the hospitals within the Group

On 30th November Air Vice Marshal T. S. Kelly, who had succeeded Colonel Watson, the first Medical Superintendent in the war years, himself retired and Mr. Williamson took over the post on a part-time basis. About this time Dr. Gregg had been replaced by Dr. I. P. Williams as Consultant Radiologist and Miss S. M. Hay had been appointed Matron in place of Miss Finch, who had left the hospital.

Dr. Morrey was one of the first pathologists in charge of the Area laboratory. He was succeeded by Dr. Whitehouse and then by Dr. J. H. Dean. In December Dr. Dean extended the work of the Area laboratory to a 24 hour service. He authorised all emergency calls and it is surprising how few of these calls there were compared to today. Theatres and X-ray also ran a 24 hour emergency service and the extra work was hard on the comparatively few staff available. Radiographers, like other technicians, were very difficult to recruit. Miss Cowper Johnson and her small staff did very well to keep the service going.

In January, 1953, interest was shown in opening a hydrotherapy pool mainly for the treatment of polio and orthopaedic patients. The billiard room in A2 Block was little used and it was proposed to attach this to the Physiotherapy Department and convert it to a hydrotherapy pool. Money was short and the work had to be paid for partly from voluntary contributions. As late as October, 1958, the Editor of the Newmarket Journal was asked to arrange an appeal to raise funds for the pool to be built. As usual the people of Newmarket rallied round and the pool was opened on 23rd July, 1960. I believe this was the first hydrotherapy pool to be opened in East Anglia. It has been extensively used and the staff pioneered the early work in this field of treatment. It is interesting that the racing industry have also built a hydrotherapy pool in the town for the treatment of racehorses.

I believe Miss Hayter was the first Superintendent Physiotherapist appointed and when she retired she was succeeded by Miss S. M. Stevens. Miss K.A.G. Sargent was appointed Assistant Superintendent Physiotherapist on lst February. Mr. E. S. Jamieson and the physiotherapists built up very high standards of treatment in this department and this remains today.

Under Miss Stevens' direction, a 16mm physiotherapy training and recruitment film was made at the hospital and used locally. It was also hired by many schools and other hospitals up and down the country and I believe is still in circulation today. The Photography Department at Addenbrooke's Hospital did all the technical work for the film and the cost of £100 was met from the Hospital Free Monies.

In the autumn of 1955 there was an outbreak of poliomyelitis in the hospital. Several contacts were found amongst the hospital staff. Those who were non-resident were sent off duty and Exning Isolation Hospital was used for the first time to isolate the contacts among the resident staff.

1956 *More Upgrading and Development*

During 1956-57 the upgrading and development of the hospital continued despite a general shortage of all grades of staff.

In January 1956, 2¼ acres of land at St. Fabians Estate was sold to the West Suffolk County Council: the present Upper School was built on this land. I recall Mr. H. R. Buck, OBE, JP, was Chairman of the Management Committee at the time. He also served as a member of the County Council and negotiated the sale.

Staff Christmas parties had always been held on a department basis and in January it was decided to change this to one Annual Ball in the town's Memorial Hall for all the staff and their guests. The Hall would only hold about 250 and since hospital staff numbered then about 300 there was always a full house and the tickets were very scarce. For the original dances a large marquee was hired to accommodate the bar and was erected alongside the main hall. Being away from the hospital a lot of prior work had to be done: the gardeners were excellent at this and we relied on them very much.

Steve Stevenson and his Band were engaged whenever possible. A charge was made for tickets and the Hospital Committee made contributions of £100 from Free Monies. The event became very popular in the town and continued for many years. On reflection, I recall, early on, one Christmas dance was held in the Drill Hall in Fordham Road, Newmarket.

In February, 1956, Miss Challice, who had done excellent work in the Group Secretary's office, retired. The number of available staffed beds was only 245: of these 63 were allocated to Diseases of the Chest.

Mr. J. S. Hesketh, the Consultant Gynaecologist, was in charge of the Maternity Unit and in order to relieve the pressure on his unit, from September, 1954, Cardigan Street Nursing Home had been used to accommodate the overflow of mothers from the hospital. It was staffed from the main unit and served a very useful purpose. As the main unit developed the need for the accommodation decreased and it was closed on 27th January, 1956, and handed back to the owners. As part of this move the local general practitioners requested a GP maternity unit of eight beds be opened above the existing hospital Maternity Unit so that they could attend their patients and use the hospital staff and facilities. Mr. Hesketh agreed and the unit was eventually opened in Ward A2 in May, 1965. There had been some talk of these units and I am sure this was one of the first to open in East Anglia. Interviews were given to Anglia television.

By March a programme to provide cubicle curtains around the patients' beds was started and the rooms above the present administrative offices in "A" Block were converted for medical staff accommodation. Miss Foster, Matron of the Exning Isolation Hospital, retired in March, 1956.

The medical beds at Addenbrooke's Hospital were under pressure and a two-way arrangement for admissions was agreed with the Newmarket General Hospital. This was possibly one of the first of the strong links the Hospital had with Addenbrooke's.

The war time corridors or covered ways, pictured below, left a lot to be desired. The movement of patients to and from the wards and theatre, X-ray, physiotherapy, etc. was very difficult in inclement weather and a start was made to enclose them in May. "C" Block was enclosed first followed by the spur from "C" Block to theatre and x-ray and, eventually, "B" Block in the summer of 1961 and later "B - C" corridor was enclosed.

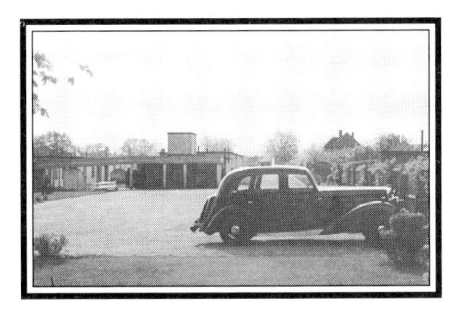

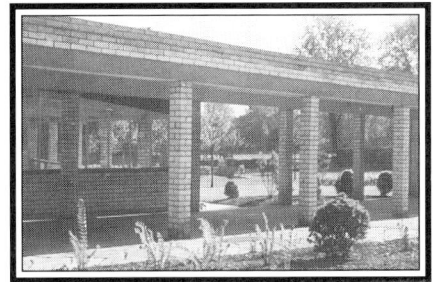

During the summer months of 1956 a Daily Living Unit was opened as part of the Occupational Therapy Department.

The Guillebaud Report on Hospital Departmental Costing had been introduced. This had shown defects and for their comparison purposes it was found necessary to accurately measure the area of all wards and departments in all the hospitals in the Group. A team of measurers was engaged under the control of the Group Treasurer and the work took months to complete.

1957 Nursing Staff Problems - Again

During 1957 the shortage of staff, particularly nursing, became acute. Out of twelve Colonial subjects recruited at Newmarket only four were still in post. A campaign to recruit nursing auxiliaries from Spain was underway. The cost of the recruits' fares to England was deducted from their salary after they had joined the hospital staff. Consideration was being given to the recruitment of nurses and midwives from New Zealand and Australia.

Through hard work a lot of foreign recruits were obtained but many of them spoke little or no English and regular language classes had to be arranged. Unfortunately most of these recruits drifted away to London in due course.

Junior medical staff were also difficult to recruit and in April, following a visit by an Inspector of the Royal College of Surgeons of England, the hospital senior house officer posts in Orthopaedic and General Surgery were recognised as qualifying training posts for the examinations for the Fellowship of the College. All other hospitals had staffing difficulties at this time.

In April the first G.P.O. mobile telephones were introduced in the TB wards. The WRVS very kindly met the cost of installation and the rental charges: this service was extended to all the wards in due course.

The temporary wartime coke stoves were still in use in the wards and consideration was being given to building a new boiler house to replace the numerous and outdated small boiler installations and the provision of a new central heating system throughout the hospital.

In June the medical staff organised a Sports Day in the paddock in "C" Block. Consideration was also being given to converting the old pharmacy into a Plaster Clinic.

In July the service lift was installed between the ground and first floor of the Maternity Unit.

The cost per patient week was reported to be £20. 5s. 2d., and the weekly allowance for provisions was reported as being exceeded by 1s. 3d. per head. One reason for this was that the patients in the TB wards were given beer and stout daily and the annual cost of this was £564. Messrs. Guinness Ltd. supplied a small amount of Guinness, free of charge, to hospitals in East Anglia. Newmarket General Hospital was a Regional Centre for meetings of various organisations and this also added to the catering costs. An example of these meetings was the clinical meetings held at Newmarket for all the Orthopaedic Surgeons of East Anglia.

In December the Matron, Miss S. M. Hay, visited Ireland for nursing recruitment. She visited six hospitals and recruited three staff nurses. The Convent of St. Louis in Newmarket helped considerably in arranging this visit. There was a local move in the town to form a Hospital League of Friends. Dr. Dorsitor was asked to negotiate on this.

Newmarket town had no public mortuary and the hospital mortuary was used on occasions. The charge made to the Urban District Council was £15 per annum and £10 per annum to the Rural District Council. This arrangement was quite common.

The chiropody service was giving trouble. Very few chiropodists were being trained and there were few practising locally who could undertake the hospital work.

It was reported to the December meeting of the Hospital Management Committee that for the past eight years the Group Engineer had arranged for three workmen to be sent from the Group Works Department at Fulbourn Hospital, for maintenance work at Newmarket General Hospital. They had been transported daily, in official time, and official transport. The cost exceeded their usefulness.

1958 *Ten Year Review*

In January, 1958, Mr. B. M. Witley was appointed Group Fire Officer, being based in "A" Block.

In May all the hospital cots were modified by the maintenance department. A number of cot deaths elsewhere had been reported and the Ministry of Health had stipulated the distance allowed between the bars of the cots.

On 21st June a garden fete and sports meeting, organised by the hospital Social Club, was held in the grounds at St. Fabians estate.

It was realised that there was an urgent need for an improved emergency electrical supply system for the boiler houses and theatres. Apart from torches and hurricane lamps there was only one battery American portable electric operating lamp available, which was kept in the theatre.

In July the Lord Lieutenant of Suffolk, the Rt. Hon. Earl of Stradbroke, presented the prizes at the Nurses' Prizegiving. He was accompanied by Countess Stradbroke. A hard tennis court was opened for the staff at St. Fabians and it was used extensively. The General Nursing Council revised the conditions of approval for General Nursing Training Schools. Amongst other things they stipulated a minimum number of 300 beds with an average occupancy of not less than 240 and 100 students in training at any one time. Unfortunately the hospital could not meet these conditions. It was considered that the abolition of the Nurses' Training School for full State Registration would have a very adverse effect upon the recruitment of nurses and consequently upon the status of the hospital. Eventually the GNC agreed to continue approval for a complete Training School for the time being.

The proposed new pharmacy in "A" Block and plaster clinic in "C" Block had been approved in principle by the Regional Hospital Board and Mr. G. Clayton Smith, a local architect, was appointed for the design work.

Ward C7 was opened as a gynaecological ward in July, 1958.

At the end of the financial year 1958 the hospital costing statistics were:

Average number of occupied beds	192
% occupation of available staffed beds	68%
Long stay cases - % of occupied beds	25%
Average stay per case - days	24
No. of cases	2,928
No. of in-patient days	70,224
No. of out-patient attendances	18,956
No. of new out-patients	5,692
Total in-patient expenditure (net)	£218,746
Total out-patient expenditure (net)	£ 39,481
In-patient cost per week	£74. 14s. 2d.

In the autumn of 1958 the Ministry of Health set up a study of the new Hospital Service which had been in operation for ten years. Considerable progress had been made in expanding the services provided for patients and upgrading the existing hospitals. In the surgical specialties the major developments were the consequences of improvements in anaesthetics and in the care before and after operation. The invention of new effective drugs and vaccines was undoubtedly the most significant area of medical advance. In these early years diphtheria was virtually eliminated as a cause of death in children. This was also true of poliomyelitis and there had been a marked drop in the death rate from tuberculosis.

In September a plan for the redecoration of wards was agreed by the Medical Staff Committee. The pending renewal of the electrical and mechanical services made this essential and a revised form of this plan is still in operation today.

There had been an outbreak of mumps and the children's ward had been in quarantine for a long time. In September the ward was divided into two equal parts to allow admissions to be resumed.

In November the 44 hour working week was introduced for the nursing and midwifery staff. There was concern over the poor standard of nurses' accommodation and it was agreed by all concerned that a new Nurses' Home was necessary.

At the end of 1958 Mr. Chappell, Catering Advisor No. 13 Group, was making recommendations for improving equipment in the main kitchen. The Consultant Advisory Services with Messrs. J. Lyons had been terminated.

The question of retention of medical records was raised again. The Ministry of Health had given some guidance in the disposal of old records. Storage space was very difficult: no conclusions were reached.

The Editor of the Newmarket Journal reported that £776 had been raised for the hospital Christmas Fund and that £1,200 was now available for the new hydrotherapy pool.

1959 *New Nurses' Home - Missed!*

Early in January, 1959, it was reported that chronic sick patients were blocking the acute beds. Many had been admitted as casualties and could not return to their homes. There was concern about the difficulty of transferring them to welfare accommodation.

At this time the Chief Pharmacist, Mr. W. Hobbs, was visiting the other hospitals in the Group and supplying drugs, etc. from the central pharmacy store. The supplies were delivered in special containers by the laundry vehicle.

In April a scheme for annual X-rays for nursing staff was introduced and this was eventually extended to all the hospital staff. It was pointed out, quite forcefully, by Miss Cowper Johnson, that the only member of the staff not X-rayed was myself tut! tut! In the same month the "Cohen Committee Report on Staphylococcal Infection in Hospitals" was published. Dr. J. H. Dean, Consultant Pathologist, was appointed Control of Infection Officer and registers of infection were introduced in all the wards and appropriate departments.

In October the Matron, Miss S. M. Hay, made a two week visit to Spain and recruited twenty trained nurses and five nursing auxiliaries.

It was reported that the cost of renewing the electrical installation was £68,065.

In December Oakfield House, which was the Calcutta Club in Old Station Road, Newmarket, was up for sale at a cost of £15,000 which included furnishings. Plans were made to purchase it for the much needed Nurses' Home. The total cost after modification to accommodate forty-five nurses was estimated to be £24,500. Due to delays it was sold to Messrs. Alpherson Caravans Ltd.

At the end of December the first Multitone pocket paging receiver system was installed and this was a great help to the telephonists who had to find senior staff quickly. The first stand-by electric generator was installed for the boiler house, theatre and portable X-ray unit. It was used in the event of power cuts or failure and the number of supply points was very limited.

1960 *Laboratory Technicians Training Scheme*

Early in 1960 a scheme to build four flats for medical staff at St. Fabians was being considered.

At the end of the financial year it was reported that the total expenditure for the hospital for the past year was £252,449.

In June there was difficulty in recruiting a hospital hairdresser. Six electric razors were purchased for use on the male wards. In the same month Oakfield House was again on the market. It was purchased for the hospital on 16th February, 1961, for the sum of £17,500. Unfortunately, the original paintings which hung on the walls down the main stairway and the chandelier were missing. Some more land at St. Fabians was sold to the West Suffolk County Council for the sum of £2,000. It was used to build police houses and a house for a District Nurse.

The Ministry of Health recommended that a Group Catering Officer should be appointed and Mr. Thorborne was the first officer to fill the post. He was based at and remained the Catering Officer for Newmarket General Hospital.

In October the RHB notified that a Regional Work Study Officer had been appointed and that a work study would be arranged for the portering staff at Newmarket General Hospital. In this month the RHB training scheme for Medical Laboratory Technicians was introduced. The training centres were the Blood Transfusion Centre, Cambridge, Papworth Hospital and Newmarket. The students had to attend each centre during the course of their training and sometimes transport was difficult.

The hospital telephone exchange was again giving trouble. The traffic had built up and complaints were being received about the delays in answering calls. A new 100 line automatic telephone exchange was installed which allowed internal calls to be dialled direct leaving the telephonist to deal with incoming and outgoing calls only. At that time the telephonist had to operate the staff call system, the fire alarm system and a number of other general duties. The night telephonists completed the hospital statistics, published the daily bed returns, which were available at 8 a.m. daily and also completed the annual SH3 statistical returns at the end of December each year.

In November Miss Welply organised the Annual Fireworks party in the Childrens' Ward. Collections were made and the parties were jolly good. Many of the childrens' families and families of hospital staff attended. The gardeners and porters helped out and it was a shame that, some years later, owing to the number of accidents, the Ministry of Health frowned on this sort of firework party and when Miss Welply left they ceased.

The County Dental Officer had been using the hospital dental clinic for a number of years for which a small charge was made. In December they provided their own health clinic in Newmarket and the arrangement ceased.

The Editor of the Newmarket Journal reported that £902. 0s. 6d. had been raised for the 1960 hospital Christmas Fund. The hospital has always been very grateful to him for this support.

1961 *Student Nurse training withdrawn*

On 9th February, 1961, six new garages were opened for the staff at St. Fabians estate.

Mr. W. Hobbs, the Group Pharmacist, was supervising the pharmaceutical work at Fulbourn Hospital: he made monthly visits.

In April Newmarket UDC held a Trades Fair on the Severals. The hospital entered a stand for nursing recruitment and much local interest was shown in it. Once again there was a general shortage of nursing staff and admissions had to be restricted.

In July there were difficulties in staffing the group laundry at Newmarket. The Nurses' Cadet Scheme had developed into a two year course for girls aged sixteen. They entered the Nurses' Training School when eighteen.

Also in July ward clerks were introduced to help the ward sisters cope with the ever-increasing amount of paper work. Initially each ward clerk served two wards but this spread to a service on all the wards as time went by.

In August Mr. Williamson retired and was replaced by Dr. Robertson, Consultant Anaesthetist, as part-time Medical Superintendent.

By October the General Nursing Council had withdrawn approval for a General Nursing Training School for student nurses but had approved a training school for enrolled nurses. This was transferred from St. Fabians to accommodation in "A" Block in the main hospital. St. Fabians house was then used as a Sisters' home. It was necessary to change the colours of the training school and hospital badge from the original white horse shoe and green bar to a green horse shoe and red bar.

The British Red Cross Society made a charge of 13s. 6d. per occupied bed for the mobile library service in the wards. This was an excellent service which was in existence for many years.

In October it was decided to include day rooms at the end of each ward.

Although this meant a loss of four beds in the wards it was a very good move and had always been appreciated by the patients. The work was completed when the electrical and mechanical services were renewed.

In November hygiene in hospital kitchens was giving concern. Dr. J. H. Dean and the Catering Officer, gave a full report to the Group Nursing Committee: most of the recommendations were implemented.

1962 *Television Coverage Again*

On 26th January, 1962, the first Annual Hospital Ball was held at Soham and Joe Loss and his band were in attendance. Mr. Eric Isaccson organised this very popular event, which raised funds, not only for the hospital but also for other hospitals in the district.

The first family planning clinic started in Newmarket in January and in March an extension between the outpatient department and the medical records department was approved.

In January a Ten Year Plan for the development of Hospitals in the No. 1 Group was published. This had little effect on Newmarket General Hospital. On 26th January, 1962, the work study on the hospital portering services was completed and their recommendations published. Shift work was introduced and a general upgrading of the service recommended. The purchase of an electric tug was recommended for delivering food trolleys to and from the wards to the main kitchen. It was used for other jobs and proved very useful.

At the end of March the Finance Officer reported that the cost of drugs was rising and the costs were constantly under review. A report was also received from the Supplies Officer on the possibility of using plastic crockery throughout the hospital. A three year controlled experiment had been completed on Ward B2. The results were not good and the costs were approximately three times that of normal earthenware crockery. No further action was taken!

By March the programme to renew the electrical and mechanical services was in full swing. This was a very difficult operation because one or two wards had to be handed over to the contractors, on a planned programme, and at the same time provide a full hospital service. The number of available beds was reduced to 237. There were only 149 patients in the hospital. At the same time the wards had to be decorated and dayrooms and other modifications made. The electrical services provided new bedhead units and the poor state of the cavity walls in "B" Block presented problems and delay in fitting these.

In April the Catering Officer introduced a patients' choice of meals system. This was the first such scheme in East Anglia and the BBC and Anglia Television service visited the hospital and interviewed the patients and staff. This type of system is common practice today. Application was made to provide a training school for apprentice cooks.

On 1st August the Chairman of the RHB, Sir Stephen Lycett Green, opened Oakfield House as a Nurses' Home. This included a tea party in the grounds and a good time was had by all.

In September White Cottage at St. Fabians was demolished to make room for the new Doctors' flats and by November two of the new medical staff flats at St. Fabians were available for occupation. At this time a start was made to introduce Vernaid disposable bed pan units in the wards.

The following main schemes were approved for when funds became available:

Upgrading Nurses' Training School	£ 7,259
Convert old pharmacy to plaster clinic	£ 7,435
Provision of "pressure Ventilation" system for theatre suite	£ 23,930
Extension to outpatient department (opened May 1964)	£ 13,390
Extension to pathology department	£ 15,100
Provision of enclosed corridor to x-ray department (work started May, 1964)	£ 12,050
Enclosure of "B - C" corridor	£ 23,950
	£103,114

When the St. Fabians estate was owned by Mr. Hammond, Mr. G. Copeman was the gardener for the estate. He lived in one of two estate cottages adjoining Exning Road and transferred to the hospital staff when the estate was purchased by the hospital. In November he retired and the two cottages and gardens were sold to the West Suffolk County Council.

By December a programme to provide the wards and departments with disposable paper sacks for refuse and soiled dressings was underway.

1963 Costs and Bed Redeployment

In January, 1963, a redeployment of hospital beds was made. Since 1948 the RHB had planned 140 general beds and beds for long stay orthopaedic, poliomyelitis and tuberculosis cases at Newmarket General Hospital. Happily these diseases had largely been mastered and there was a need for the redeployment of beds which would provide a bed complement of 276, including 60 geriatric, 132 maternity and other specialist beds associated with the new Teaching Hospital at Cambridge and District General Hospital at Bury St. Edmunds.

The main scheme costing at Newmarket General Hospital showed that the low bed occupancy was an overriding factor in the high cost, viz

Year	Bed Complement	Average Occupancy
1949	450	204
1950	450	213
1951	450	220
1952	450	210
1953	375	210
1954	374	197
1955	330	206
1956	338	190
1957	338	189
1958	339	183
1959	326	165
1960	326	157
1961	326	150

Under the main costing scheme Newmarket General Hospital was classed as "mainly acute". This was because of the long stay TB patients and geriatric patients who had arrived. There were only one or two other hospitals of this type in East Anglia and it was therefore difficult to get a proper comparison of costs with other hospitals. Control of expenditure to annual estimates was much to the fore at this time. In February the Ministry of Health advisors visited the hospital and made a report on the hospital domestic services and in July the RHB work study team also studied the domestic services.

The new boiler house in "C" Block was built in January but, unfortunately, did not include the new maintenance workshop buildings. It was previously mentioned that the money for these had been spent on wall tiles for upgrading the main kitchen.

There were no waiting lists of any consequence at this time.

In February a request was received from the Newmarket UDC for food to be cooked in the hospital kitchen for "Meals on Wheels". The hospital was not able to help at this time but did provide a service at a later date.

In the spring of 1963 a "no smoking" rule was enforced in the wards and corridors. Notices to this effect were displayed everywhere and the hospital became a much better place for it.

A Group Almoner, based at Newmarket General Hospital, was appointed.

On 30th June Mr. H. E . Merrin, the Superintendent Engineer for both the No. 1 and No. 13 Groups retired. He was succeeded by Mr. H. Holtz. The post of Building Supervisor for the two Groups was created: he was based at Newmarket.

The nursing staff had objected to counting ward linen for indenting and inventory check purposes and in June the counting of linen ceased. The linen racks in the wards and departments were marked to predetermined levels and the laundry staff topped up the linen to these levels daily. Stocks from the central linen store were delivered to the wards in large, purpose made, linen trolleys. Control was based on issues made from the central linen store.

At this time the first mention was made of centralizing all the laundry services into an Area laundry for the No. 1 and No. 13 Groups at Fulbourn Hospital.

In July Francis Pym, MC, MP, attended the Annual Nurses' Prizegiving and presented the prizes.

Dr. W. Davison was the Consultant in charge of the geriatric wards in "B" Block and a move was made to open a much larger geriatric unit at Newmarket with the appointment of an extra geriatrician. In August application was made for a licence for an Enrolled Nurses' Training School in place of the present Preliminary General Nurses' Training School. This was eventually agreed.

The electrical contract was completed in November and by this time the new central heating system was in operation. Some difficulties arose with the central heating and modifications had to be in "A" and "B" Blocks. The Ministry of Health Building Notes (No. 4) stated that the temperature in the wards should be 65 degrees F. and the system had been set up for this temperature. The nursing staff would not accept this and I do not think the temperature was ever agreed locally. Whenever possible radiators were positioned under windows in the wards and Mr. Allison, the Hospital Engineer, was always complaining that the nursing staff were opening the windows to remove nasty smells and then complaining that the temperature in the ward was low. Such is hospital life.

There was a shortage of midwives and they were hired from an agency just to keep the service running. This was a last resort and the approval of the Ministry of Health to use the agency had to be sought. Non-practicing midwives, who were married or retired, etc., were written to in the hope that they would return and help out.

In December Dr. Gairdner, the Consultant Paediatrician from Addenbrooke's Hospital, requested a "Mother and Child Unit" to be opened at the end of Ward C3.

1964 *Work Studies*

In January, 1964, car parking was presenting a real problem and the work study team recommended part of the paddock be turned into a car park. This was eventually done. I recall that in the early 1950's the problem had been to supply sufficient spaces for bicycles and it is interesting how quickly the problem changed to car parks. Every hospital has it.

In April disposable hypodermic needles were introduced throughout the hospital.

By July the hospital bed complement was:

General Medicine	43
Gynaecology	8
Ophthalmic	6
Diseases of the Chest	18
Geriatrics	33
General Surgery	26
Ear, Nose and Throat	6
Orthopaedic	42
Maternity	15
Oral Surgery	5
	202

On 30th September the hospital Church of England Chaplain, Rev. Malachi retired. He was succeeded by the Rev. Edmundson. Shortly afterwards the use of the hospital Church was under dispute.

In November a physiotherapy clinic was opened in the health centre at Haverhill, staffed from the hospital physiotherapy department. Public transport between Newmarket and Haverhill was difficult.

In the autumn the cost of providing furniture for the new ward day rooms was £882. Our old friend the Newmarket Journal Christmas Fund paid part of this.

In December the work study report on the hospital domestic service was received. The main recommendations were:

1. a Domestic Superintendent be appointed.

2. a central mechanical crockery washup unit be opened close to the main kitchen.

3. mobile cleaning teams be formed for programme cleaning of the wards and departments.

4. mechanical scrubbing and polishing machines be purchased for the use of the cleaning teams.

The report recommendations were eventually implemented and with it came considerable change. The departmental heads and ward sisters were relieved of the responsibility for domestic cleaning and the entire service came under the central control of the hospital Domestic Superintendent. Apart from the daily cleaning, the main cleaning was done by mechanised mobile teams on a planned basis and a high standard of cleaning was obtained. The cost of the new service was considerable and the RHB would only fund service schemes of this nature after a work study report had been received. The Regional Works Study Officer was Mr. Arthur Hulme who proved to be a very good friend to Newmarket General Hospital.

As time went by work studies were carried out on the hospital telephone exchange, the medical records department, the catering department and the portering services. They obtained a considerable amount of money and there is no doubt that they raised the standards in all of these departments.

Unfortunately, all the studies were done at different dates with the consequence that interdepartmental flexibility, which is so important, ceased. The studies recommended quite separate bonus schemes for each department which destroyed the old type of flexibility. A few examples are:

The day time telephonists were always very busy but, generally speaking, the male night telephonists whose shift was from 9 p.m. to 8 a.m. were slack. With the exception of emergencies the hospital was quiet during the hours of the night shift and for many years the night telephonists kept the statistical records of the hospital. They received reports from the wards and prepared the daily bed states which were delivered to the appropriate department by 8 a.m. each day. They kept the daily admissions and discharges book which had to agree with the bed states and other records appertaining to patients' statistics. They also completed the annual SH3 returns required by the Ministry of Health. They were interested in their work and were valuable members of the staff. Two long serving night telephonists were Mr. F. Milne and Mr. K. Ronald.

I have always had a high opinion of hospital gardening staff. Their work is seasonal and they work hard during the summer months and take a pride in their work. After the trees have been pruned in the autumn there is not enough inside work to keep all the gardening staff occupied during the winter months. Those who could be spared formed a team with the male operators of the domestic services and washed down the walls of the wards. The work was programmed and the walls in all the wards were cleaned once a year. I always thought they liked doing a useful job during the slack winter months. The work study on the domestic services stopped this.

The two hospital storekeepers for the provisions and general stores worked for years as a team and acted as relief for each other during holidays or sickness. Mr. Fred Symonds was considered the senior since the general store was very much larger and he enjoyed a higher rate of pay. The work study included the provision storekeeper in the catering staff bonus scheme so that his wages were higher than Fred Symonds in the general store. Fred was very annoyed and I didn't blame him.

The work study teams did obtain monies from the RHB, which the individual hospitals could never have obtained, but it was very difficult to get the officer back to correct errors and mistakes. The hospital administration had no authority to do this and it was a strong opinion that it would have been much better if the work study team had been instructed to do one study on all the ancillary staff and introduce a common bonus scheme.

In industry work study is a local service and is used in a different way. It can be called on at short notice. When used on a regional basis the long periods of waiting for a study and the delays in formal reports and Committee meetings is not good and if local management cannot make sensible changes the advantages are limited. I understand the work study service has now been considerably improved.

Nursing

In 1964 the hospital nurses and nursing were very much under review. The Royal College of Nursing published "A Reform of Nurse Education", familiarly known as the "Platt Report" after the committee chairman, Sir Harry Platt. The Platt report and its successor, the "Briggs" report, were not put into operation at this time. Two years after "Platt" came the "Salmon" report, properly entitled "The Report of the Committee on Senior Nursing Staff Structure" and, again, universally referred to by the Chairman's name. The implementation of this report which happened in many hospitals soon afterwards radically altered the traditional nursing staff structure.

At risk to life and limb I feel I must mention a few more names of long serving members of the nursing staff who will be well remembered. Unfortunately it is not possible to mention them all.

In the early days, the first Matron was Mrs. V. Minter, followed by Mrs. A. V. Heasman, who was Matron from 1912 until she retired in 1942. Mrs. Heasman was followed by Miss Lithgow, who was the Matron of the EMS Hospital during the war years. When Miss Lithgow retired, Miss Finch was appointed Matron for a short time, followed by Miss S. M. Hay. Many people will remember Matron Hay, as she was known, and the high standards she set and insisted upon. Miss Finegan succeeded Miss Hay on her retirement: she was the last of the Matrons and became the first Senior Nursing Officer when the new Salmon structure was implemented in 1967. Some other long serving members of the nursing staff that come to mind are:

Ward C8	Sister Cudden, Sister Bowyer, Mrs. Alice Atkinson
Ward C9	Sister Hayward
Ward B6 and Day Hospital	Sister Wedgewood
Outpatients	Sister Brisco

Ward B4	Sister Skipp
Ward C3	Sister Claydon
Ward A1	Sister White
Ward B2	Mr. Caunt, Sister Farahty
Theatre	Sister Rolfe, Staff Nurse Lyles, Mr. Bastin, Sister Kingswell, Mr. Leo Maycock.
Night Superintendent	Mrs. Macklin
Sister Tutor	Miss Meredith, Sister Parr
Assistant Matrons	Miss Sarbutt, who acted as Matron for a time, Miss Ford and Miss Brown and, of course, the
Home Sister	Miss Cleghorn, will be well remembered.

The recommendations of the "Salmon" report were implemented in 1967 and the first Senior Nursing Officer to be appointed was Miss Finegan, who was succeeded by Miss M. Armstrong. There is no doubt that with the introduction of "Salmon" there came a new outlook on nursing and, dare I say it, the old image of the strict Matron and Ward Sister disappeared and the hospital nursing service became much more flexible and, in my view, the team work with all the other hospital departments was improved. Miss Penney followed Miss Armstrong and when she retired Miss Bowyer, who was the ward sister on Ward C8 and Nursing Officer for "B" Block, became the hospital Service Nursing Officer. Miss Bowyer was followed by Miss A. Dunachie who is the Nursing and Patient Services Manager today.

The implementation of the "Salmon" report radically altered the traditional staff structure. In the general hospitals nursing had been an almost exclusively female occupation, the head of the service being the Matron. Below came the Deputy, Assistants and Sisters or Charge Nurses. It was such a small structure that a nurse with ambitions above ward nursing either waited for dead (or retired) women's shoes or changed hospitals frequently to get promotion. Either way it was often a frustrating experience. The "Salmon" report recommended a more elaborate staff structure by suggesting that the positions of Matrons should be abolished. In their place would be Head of Nursing Services, either a man or woman, below that, Senior Nursing Officers, Nursing Officers and below them Sisters or Charge Nurses. The Nursing Officers and upwards were purely in an administrative capacity and were to receive training as such. This was quite enough to produce considerable muttering amongst the staff on the lines of Chiefs and Indians. It involved male nurses much more in the service. "Parkinson's Law" says that a committee will argue fiercely over the allocation of paper clips but will cheerfully agree to the expenditure of £1m. In the same way hospital nursing staff, usually so resistant to the smallest change, accepted this radical alteration with surprisingly little fuss.

Hospital administration was also changing. "Functional management" was slowly introduced: this meant that Group officers were appointed to be responsible for the services in all the hospitals in the Group. Apart from Nursing these were for Catering, Domestic, Personnel, Fire, Engineering, Medical Records, Buildings and Pharmacy.

Most of these services had always been the responsibility of the Hospital Secretary and while, at Newmarket General Hospital, the Group Secretary was also the Hospital Secretary, the new system worked in a confused sort of way.

1965 *Extra beds*

In January, 1965, the County Medical Officer of Health for West Suffolk, submitted a report on the standard of hygiene in the catering department. Such reports were made from time to time and were always welcomed. Whenever possible the recommendations were implemented.

In the same month, Mr. E. S. Jamieson, Consultant Orthopaedic Surgeon, was given clinical sessions at Addenbrooke's Hospital, Cambridge. Newmarket General Hospital had always enjoyed ties with Addenbrooke's and a number of their consultant medical staff held outpatient clinics and had an allocation of beds in the wards at Newmarket Hospital.

In March three medical students were attached to the hospital from Addenbrooke's. As the Medical School grew in Cambridge more and more students were attached to the main hospitals in the Region.

Mr. J. Burton was appointed hospital Catering Officer in April and Miss Mary Finegan was appointed Matron on 14th June.

In April a few members of the House Committee visited Copthorne Hospital and on their return recommended a central wash up unit be installed. This was part of the work study report and would avoid each ward staff having to wash crockery and containers after each meal. In May the work study report on the domestic services had been received and the recommendations were being implemented. The post of Domestic Superintendent was advertised and a contract made with the New Chesterton Window Cleaning Co. Ltd., for annual ward and department wall washing.

The Hospital Staff Association held a very good garden party at Oakfield House in June. They hired a marquee for the purpose and a good time was had by all. Also in June, the old pig sty near the Field Road entrance was demolished and a car park for twelve cars provided at the end of "B" Block.

At this time it was agreed that there was a need for more female geriatric beds and that another ward should be opened as soon as the nursing staff were available. The residents in Linton Close complained about the poor condition of the hospital boundary wall, which formed part of the maintenance department workshops. The workshops were also in a bad state of repair and it was agreed that alternative accommodation should be found for them as soon as possible.

The Ministry of Health approved the sale of Exning Isolation Hospital and it was put up for public auction by D. L. January on 21st July. It did not reach the reserve price but was sold at a later date.

It was reported that the new occupational therapy department was functioning well and that the advertisements for pupil nurses in the Irish newspapers had not been successful. Ways of improving the hospital catering service were being considered. A team of nursing, medical and administrative staff went to see a central plated meal tray service which was in being at Ipswich Hospital. It was thought to be ideal but the cost of implementation was, unfortunately, out of the question at the time. A similar system is used in most large hospitals today.

In July a proposal to establish a much larger Area laundry at Fulbourn Hospital was promoted but the RHB did not agree at the time, although the scheme was introduced later.

The annual inventory check for 1965 showed a deficiency of £21. 11s. 6d. and a surplus of £4. 12s. 11d. In August Ward C7 was being upgraded. A nursing liaison scheme with Addenbrooke's Hospital was introduced.

Mr. T. H. Todd was the first Domestic Supervisor appointed in September. In the same month the closure of the Ipswich railway passenger line at Newmarket was being considered: it was thought the closure would have little effect on the hospital.

The RHB had agreed to the proposed mother and child unit for Ward C3, although funds for the work involved were not available at this time. In October the priority order for the hospital capital works programme was:

Improvements to theatre including upgrading ancillary rooms and providing pressure ventilation	£28,050
Improvements to physiotherapy department	£ 4,750
Improvements to occupational therapy and daily living facilities	£ 2,750
Improved accommodation for maternity unit	(plans not yet agreed)
Enclosure of main "B - C" corridor	£23,950

Towards the end of 1965 a campaign was held to persuade trained nursing staff, who had married or retired, to return to nursing at the hospital. This was called "the Back to Nursing campaign" and received a very good response locally. Miss Diana Wilson was the first trainee cook to be appointed under the Assistant Cook's Training Scheme. She was seconded to Addenbrooke's Hospital for a short period as part of her training.

Hopes were high of bringing Ward C5 and C7 into use and also to opening Ward B3 as an extra female geriatric ward. The Ministry of Health, in their circular HM(65)71, gave guidance on the retention of medical records and hoped this would be implemented by Hospital Authorities not later than March, 1968. The medical staff did not agree!

1966 Laundry Closes

In January, 1966, the Newmarket Round Table presented the hospital with an electric ripple bed, which was the most up to date method of preventing bed sores.

In December a team of youngsters from the Forest School Camp were attached to the hospital. They demolished the dangerous air raid shelters in "B" Block and did landscape gardening under the directions of Bill Hazard, who was the head gardener at the time. Their work was voluntary.

By December the Area laundry at Fulbourn Hospital had been opened and the hospital laundry, which had given a good service since the original Workhouse was built, was closed.

1967 Hospitals Regrouping

The RHB had submitted proposals to the Ministry of Health for regrouping the hospitals in the western part of the East Anglia region and they were approved on 1st June, 1967. Part of the proposals were that the South West (No. 1) Group should be disbanded and the hospitals in it be moved into other Hospital Management Committee Groups. The Newmarket General Hospital was attached to the West Suffolk Hospital Management Committee (HMC) in Bury St. Edmunds, rather like the attachment in the 1930's.

In March the hospital was participating in a scheme for medical graduates from overseas coming to the UK for further training. Four places were allocated to the hospital and the graduates were required to be resident. At this time the recruitment of physiotherapists was difficult as well and the hospital was fortunate in obtaining the services of Miss Dunston from Burwell, on a part-time basis, to run the Haverhill Physiotherapy Clinic.

Block "A" kitchen, which had been used as a store, was converted into an ancillary staff changing room. A patient from the Soham area, who had been involved in a road accident, was transferred by helicopter to Stoke Mandeville Hospital for specialized treatment. The playing fields at the Upper School, opposite the hospital, had been designated as a landing ground for helicopters as part of the "Major Incident" scheme.

The plans for extending the maternity unit were still under discussion and the General Nursing Council became involved.

The last meeting of the South West (No. 1) Group HMC was held in the hospital Board Room on 21st March, 1967. Mr. A. W. Youngs became the Regional Training Officer and the members of his staff were found other posts. The Supplies Department moved to Fulbourn Hospital and, gradually, the Finance Department was run down, the staff being transferred to the No. 13 Group at Fulbourn Hospital or to the West Suffolk HMC at Bury St. Edmunds. Mr. G. Meadowcroft, the Finance Officer, retired in May, 1972. Mr. R. W. Heasman became Hospital Secretary at Newmarket General Hospital and the hospital functioned independently of the Group departments which had been based on the premises.

Chapter Nine

WEST SUFFOLK HOSPITAL MANAGEMENT COMMITTEE

1967 *New Management*

The first meeting of the West Suffolk HMC, after Newmarket General Hospital had joined the Group, was held at the Group headquarters in Bury St. Edmunds on 30th May, 1967. Mr. M. D. Corke was in the Chair and Mr. P. M. Cooke was the Group Secretary. The officers of the old No. 1 Group and members of the Hospital House Committee were invited to attend.

In April an automatic beverage vending machine was installed in "C" Block. The Newmarket Round Table kindly agreed to meet the cost of three months' rental.

The Report of the GNC Inspection, made in November, 1966, was received. The recommendations included:

(a) the nursing staff should be relieved of sluicing foul linen on the wards.

(b) the height of the wash basins in the Childrens' Ward be lowered for crippled children and that one adult toilet be replaced by a special child's toilet.

The GNC also recommended that the hospital be provisionally approved as a Training School for the Roll (for enrolled nurses), subject to the sluice room in the maternity unit being upgraded.

Although recruitment of physiotherapists was difficult the medical staff insisted that weekend cover by the department was essential.

Since the resignation of Mrs. Lamport Smith, the hospital almoner, some time earlier, Mrs. I. Bell had assumed the duties and it was reported that she had done excellent work in keeping the department going, single handed. She continued in the role until the department was taken over by the Social Services in 1974.

On 25th May the hospital nursing staff float gained third place in the Soham Town Carnival.

On 30th June Mrs. E. Mason, who was then the Assistant Group Catering

Officer, retired. As a member of the catering service she had served the hospital for twenty-five years. She attended the last meeting of the No. 1 Group HMC and was thanked for her loyal services.

In June, too, the mother and child unit in Ward C3 was opened. This was another first for Newmarket and Anglia television were present at the opening. Unfortunately one mother, living in the Fordham area, was not aware that she and her child would be on television and I spent a long time tracing her for her permission. This was reluctantly given.

Lieut. Colonel Ruth Fussell, U.S.A.F. Nursing Officer, presented the prizes at the annual Nurses' Prize Giving.

Another local "Back to Nursing" campaign, to recruit nurses for the ophthalmic and professorial surgical wards, due to be opened in "C" Block, was held between 9th and 13th October, with quite a good response.

In August the first Hospital Joint Staff Consultative Committee was formed. In September the sewing room was moved to new premises in the new central linen room and on 18th September Mr. J. V. Burton was appointed Group Catering Officer: Miss Jenkins succeeded him as Hospital Catering Officer.

Contacts had been made in Hong Kong for the recruitment of nursing staff.

In December the upgrading of the theatre suite commenced. The staff recreation room in "C" Block was adapted as a temporary theatre and an expensive Octatent purchased as a temporary theatre. In practice this was not satisfactory and all credit is due to the surgeons and theatre staff in keeping the hospital service going under very difficult conditions.

Mr. A. S. Kent, Chairman of the Hospital House Committee, kindly gave a bottle of champagne for the best decorated ward for Christmas. This was won by Ward B2 and was enjoyed to the full by staff!

1968 *Ophthalmic Surgery Arrives*

On 19th January, 1968, the Supplies Department moved from Ward B5 into the new Area Supplies Department at Fulbourn Hospital. Ward B5 was now available for geriatric patients.

In February, a scheme was arranged for Enrolled Nurses training with secondment from Addenbrooke's to Newmarket General Hospital. The first group consisted of six pupil nurses. This month also saw an informal arrangement made with the Students Appointments Officer of the University College Hospital, London, to provide a steady supply of approved graduates to fill pre-registration medical posts in the hospital. Dr. Arden Jones was the negotiator.

Members of the House Committee in 1968 were Mr. A. S. Kent, Mrs. O'Callaghan, Mr. H. R. Buck, OBE, Mrs. G. B. Barling, Mr. E. W. Bullman, Mr. R. F. A. Clark, the Hon. Mrs. E. McKenna and Mr. A. S. C. Gibson, JP.

On 8th April Ward C5 was opened as a mixed sex ophthalmic ward for Mr. J. Cairns and Mr. J. Watson, Consultant Ophthalmologists at Addenbrooke's Hospital. Their waiting lists had built up and the use of the ward was necessary until their new ophthalmic unit was built at that hospital. The trained nursing staff travelled daily to and from Cambridge and Newmarket provided the nursing auxiliaries and other non-nursing staff. The ward did excellent work and a very happy relationship prevailed with Addenbrooke's who also held ophthalmic outpatient clinics at the hospital for many years. Miss Perris Taylor, Ophthalmologist, had used a number of beds and had outpatient clinics at the hospital.

During April all staff tea breaks, morning and afternoon, were centralised in the staff restaurant. A number of other arrangements had previously been tried: nursing staff had had to use the ward kitchens and the junior in the office made the tea without other staff stopping work. The new arrangement meant the ten-minute break extended to twenty minutes since the restaurant was some way from the wards and offices and shifts and day work was interrupted.

The Ministry of Health agreed to purchase 23 Field Terrace Road. The house was located close to the hospital and was used to accommodate married medical staff.

In May a ward and department linen and general supplies topping-up system was introduced. The ward sister and departments were no longer responsible for their stocks of linen, cleaning materials, etc.

The General Nursing Council approved a scheme for training part-time Enrolled Nurses. Mr. W. Long, the Head Porter, resigned after eighteen years' hospital service.

A working party on a Group Major Incident scheme had prepared a draft report and this was being considered.

In August the BBC 2 television programmes were available and Radio Rentals reported that there was ample signal strength for the ward sets to receive the programmes. Our friends, the Newmarket Journal Fund, paid for some television sets to be replaced and for a new aerial system to receive the new BBC 2 programme.

Work was in progress to convert Ward B5 into a female geriatric ward and this was opened on 16th June, 1969. The central dish wash-up unit was opened in "C" Block on 7th October, 1968, Messrs. Hobarts' technical advisor instructing staff in its use.

In October the first recommendation to use microwave ovens for cooking meals for night staff was made. Mr. J. Pountain, who had been the hospital dentist for a number of years, resigned on 31st October.

On 1st November the hospital laundry service was transferred from Fulbourn Hospital to the new Area laundry at Bury St. Edmunds. Repairs to linen and articles of clothing were done centrally.

In November, too, the local jockeys offered to raise funds to purchase a mini bus for the hospital. A dance to raise funds for this was held in the Memorial Hall, Newmarket, in February, 1969.

A nasty infection occurred in the Ophthalmic ward C5. The RHB set up a control of infection committee to investigate and identify the possible cause. Both the ward and temporary theatre were closed and the ward did not reopen until 27th January, 1969.

In October work started on improving the maternity unit and the unit was moved to Ward C4 whilst the contractors' work was in progress. During the autumn the first attempt was made to recruit an unpaid voluntary organiser.

1969 *The First Transplant*

The contractors working on upgrading the theatre suite completed their work and the theatres reopened on 27th January, 1969.

In February an assisted staff transport service was started for the nursing staff living in the Haverhill area since public transport was not available.

Dr. W. Davison requested a day hospital unit be provided for the geriatric patients in "B" Block and visits were made to other hospitals where these units were in operation.

Mrs. A . T. Murray was acting Matron from 31st March, 1969, retiring on 30th November, 1970.

On 8th April the professorial surgical ward C4 was opened. As part of the upgrading an extension had been built between Ward C4 and C5 to provide extra sluicing, toilets and bathing facilities, etc. The two wards looked like this:

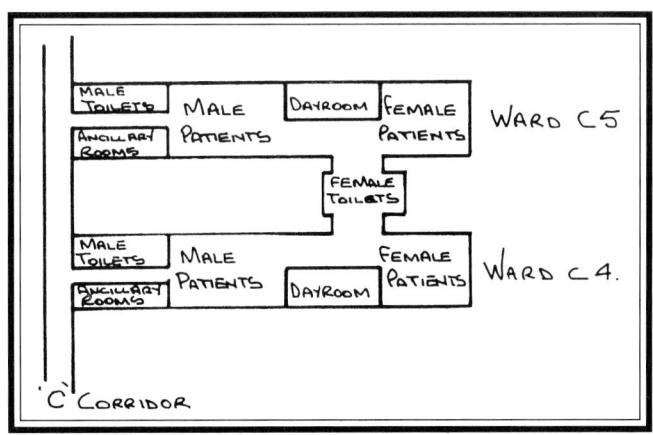

```
                MALE
                TOILETS   MALE      DAYROOM  FEMALE
                ANCILLARY PATIENTS           PATIENTS    WARD C5
                ROOMS
                                    FEMALE
                                    TOILETS

                MALE
                TOILETS   MALE               FEMALE
                ANCILLARY PATIENTS  DAYROOM  PATIENTS    WARD C4.
                ROOMS

          'C' CORRIDOR
```

They were both mixed sex wards, which was unusual at that time. Both male and female patients used the common day room and shared the same feeding arrangements. The new extensions, however, provided separate toilet and bathing facilities for female patients.

A young boy had been admitted, following a road accident, and was a hopeless case. He was being kept alive on a life support machine and Mr. E. S . Jamieson, the Consultant Orthopaedic Surgeon, notified Professor Sir Roy Calne that the boy's relatives had agreed to his organs being used for transplant purposes. Professor Calne decided to do a liver transplant operation and requested that he could do this in the upgraded theatres at Newmarket General Hospital. The arrangement was that the specialized, trained nursing staff would be sent, daily, from the Transplant Centre in Cambridge and the nursing auxiliaries and ancillary staff would be provided by Newmarket. The County

Coroner at Bury St. Edmunds was consulted and gave his permission for the removal of the organ but it was not until 4 p.m. on 7th April that the arrangements between the two hospitals were agreed.

The normal day's operation lists were in progress and did not finish until about 6 p.m. The theatre staff then had to prepare the theatres for the transplant operation. Mr. Bastin, the Theatre Superintendent, was attending a Middle Management Course at Ipswich and was recalled to the hospital by telephone. Extra sterilizing and blood had to be obtained from Bury St. Edmunds and there was much to do in a short time.

Mrs. Winnie Smith, who I believe lived in Welwyn Garden City, was the recipient. She walked into the female surgical ward opposite Ward C4 at about 7 p.m. and was given her pre-op treatment there. Professor Calne and his team, together with all their equipment, arrived at about 8 p.m. and after a quick meal with the Newmarket staff, started the transplant operation at about 10 p.m. It was finished in the early hours of 8th April, 1969. Quite a few people came from Cambridge to see the operation and I recall one lady who had come to this country from overseas to learn about transplants. She was very keen. The hospital staff were also present, some participating, and the theatres were pretty full.

There was some difficulty in accommodating Mrs. Smith in the surgical ward and when Professor Calne arrived he suggested she should be the first patient in his new ward C4. This meant that part of the ward had to be prepared for occupation whilst the operation was in progress. The Hospital Engineer and Domestic Superintendent were recalled to the hospital to clean the ward and switch on and test the services. Stocks of clean linen, etc. were obtained from the central linen store and pharmacy. Mr. Swann, the GPO engineer who did most of the telephone work at the hospital, was traced and left his local public house to connect the ward to the hospital telephone exchange. I received a really good rocket from the GPO for this dastardly deed!

Following the operation Mrs. Smith was accommodated in the new ward, as the first patient, and I was told she was sitting up in bed over a cup of coffee at about 8 a.m. the next morning. She stayed on the ward for about eight days and was then transferred to Professor Calne's transplant unit in Cambridge.

In those days it was most unusual for a transplant operation of this nature, to be carried out outside of the transplant centre. In fact, comparatively few liver transplants had been done. I was told that Professor Calne wanted to show that it was possible for his team to do this away from his centre. The senior staff were concerned that knowledge of this unusual operation should not leak to the national press and it was agreed between the local medical, nursing and administrative staff that only essential staff should be told and certainly no one outside the hospital. The Group HQ at Bury St. Edmunds were told two days after the operation and were very upset at not being put in the picture from the start. We were unpopular for a long time! Secrecy had to be maintained and shortly before Mrs. Smith left the hospital the Coroner informed us that a member of the press had asked him to confirm that he had given permission for the boy's organs to be removed. He had no alternative but to confirm this and shortly afterwards all hell was let loose.

The inquest on the boy was held in the hospital Board Room, which was full to capacity. Prior to this the Coroner told us that a person would attend who said he had evidence that the operation was a case of murder and he intended to prove it at the inquest. Dr. A. W. Robertson, the hospital Consultant Anaesthetist, had switched off the life support machine and he had to attend the inquest. He was very distressed. However, the inquest was interesting, but uneventful, and the hospital soon settled down to routine work again. It was quite an experience and I understand that Mrs. Winnie Smith returned to work and proved to be the longest living liver transplant patient of her day.

In April an urgent request was received from the medical staff for a recovery/intensive care unit to be built alongside the theatres.

On 23rd April a one-day "Teach In " for Chaplains in the District was arranged at the hospital. Only about six were expected and to our surprise twenty-five attended. They all had a healthy appetite and the day was a great success. This was the first meeting of its kind and later they were held on a Group basis at Bury St. Edmunds.

On 30th April Mr. Fred Milne, the night telephonist for the past twenty-three years, retired. Miss Jessie Cockleton, Dining Room assistant, also retired after twenty-two years' service. On 3rd May a 21st anniversary party for the Nurses' Training School was held.

In May, the former Tramps' Wards and wartime decontamination centre were demolished and the area redesigned: this is now the entrance to the hospital. It was reported that there had been a general increase in the work load in all the departments of the hospital. The bed complement at this time was 285.

In August the Major Accident Plan for the hospitals in the Group was agreed. This also involved the local police, ambulance and other local services and also included a hospital staff recall system, separate from the telephone exchange. Regular exercises were held to test the plan.

Sister L. M. Rowe, Night Superintendent, retired on 31st August. In the same month the General Nursing Council Inspector of Training Schools recommended that permanent approval be given to the Newmarket General Hospital as a Training School for the Roll. This was indeed good news.

On 27th September Mrs. V. Ranner, who had been the sewing room superintendent for twenty-seven years, retired. She had given excellent service and a jolly good party was held in the sewing room. Miss M. Finegan retired from the post of Matron on 16th December and was succeeded by Miss M. Armstrong who became the Senior Nursing Officer with the introduction of the "Salmon" report. Miss L. Macklin was appointed Night Superintendent on 1st October.

On 1st October a "pay as you eat" service for all staff was introduced in the staff restaurant. Previously, resident staff had had a deduction made from their salary for meals. In the same month a new plan for all the hospital car parks was agreed.

The future Christmas arrangements were reconsidered in 1969 and a number of changes made, viz

(a) it had been the practice for most of the local churches and other organisations to send carol parties to the hospital just before Christmas. The nursing staff traditionally toured the wards singing carols on Christmas Eve. This was thought too much for the patients and the churches were asked to send one carol party combining all the church choirs. The schools also sent parties of school children to the hospital and they were also asked to send one combined party in future years.

(b) for many years members of the House Committee, with senior staff, had toured the hospital wards on Christmas morning. This was an official visit and it interrupted the ward arrangements. The visit was cancelled.

(c) it was agreed that wards should be combined as far as possible to allow as many patients as possible to be sent home and the maximum number of nursing staff to enjoy Christmas at home with their families.

(d) it had always been the practice for each ward to have a whole turkey, carved by the consultant in charge of the ward, followed by a party in the side wards. This was no longer practical when the wards were condensed and therefore the turkeys were carved in the catering department for all the open wards. The geriatric wards, where the numbers were high, continued to receive whole turkeys. The new system was flexible and proved to be a much better arrangement.

Towards the end of the year the mobile telephone service was extended to Ward B1 and B2. Mr. S. N. Neville from Saffron Walden kindly met the cost of installation and of one year's rental. Mr. Neville owned a wonderful fairground steam engine and steam organ. He visited many events and included a collecting box for the hospital on the steam engine. He made other gifts from the proceeds.

At this time the recruitment of nursing staff had improved and there was a shortage of residential accommodation for them. There was no help from the Urban District Council.

1970 *"Salmon" introduced*

In February, 1970, the Jockey Association of Great Britain met the cost of £465 for a water purification unit for the hydrotherapy pool and the presentation was made at a sherry party held in the Physiotherapy Department. In the same month there was a very bad epidemic of influenza. Although no wards were closed there were very few nursing staff on the wards and many voluntary workers helped out. A letter of thanks, signed by the Chairman of the Hospital Committee, was sent to all members of the nursing staff.

On 16th March a limited central sterile supply service (C.S.S.D.) was introduced for the hospital wards and departments. The service was provided by the new Area C.S.S.D. at the West Suffolk Hospital, Bury St. Edmunds, and as the service increased the old steam kettle sterilizer, which had been the main form of sterilizing, was no longer used. Sterilized sealed packs of both instruments and dressings were being provided in all hospitals and with it came another problem in the form of a little devil called the "Pharaoh Ant".

This minute little chap had lived happily in many hospitals, including ours, since time began. He had no effect on the steam sterilizer but it was found he could get into the sealed packs and when found there the contents of the pack could no longer be used. The ants were found in the maternity ward, theatre and in some of the general wards and appeared to live happily in the main service ducts in "C" corridor.

Outside contractors were engaged to spray the ducts and paint a line of ant killer about one foot from the floor round all the walls in the wards and departments throughout the hospital. This was very expensive and one day when the contractors were spraying ducts in "C" Block the spray came out one end and looked like smoke. The sister in the outpatient department immediately pushed the fire alarm button and when the fire brigade arrived what was thought to be smoke was still filling the corridor. They put their water hose down one end of the duct and a very wet and disgruntled member of the contractors' staff came out the other end holding his, still hot, spray gun. It was a problem and may still be so today. Miss Beeson, from the Ministry of Agriculture and Fisheries in Cambridge, was the advisor and she admitted very little was known about the ant at that time. The theatres at Papworth Hospital were closed for a long time because of the Pharaoh Ant.

On 5th March a meeting was held to discuss the voluntary work in the hospital with all the voluntary organisations involved. Forty-seven representatives attended and it was agreed a Voluntary Organiser should be appointed as soon as possible. Unfortunately, at this time, these posts were very demanding and unpaid.

From April, the ward above the maternity unit was used as a staff sick bay.

Dr. I. P. Williams, Consultant Radiologist, left the hospital on 1st July and Miss K. Armstrong was appointed Senior Nursing Officer on the same day. A patients' satisfaction study was held in July and it was nice to know that this was quite satisfactory at Newmarket General Hospital.

In October Dr. J. B. Ewan, MD, DPH, Senior Medical Officer to the RHB, presented the prizes at the annual Hospital Prizegiving.

In November Dr. A. W. Robertson retired and the post of Medical Superintendent ceased. The Chairman of the Medical Staff Committee, the Senior Nursing Officer and the Hospital Secretary met once a week to discuss and agree the day to day work of the hospital. This arrangement worked very well.

Towards the end of 1970 the Nursing Officers were appointed as part of the "Salmon" structure. They were;

Miss Roddy - formerly Assistant Matron, appointed Nursing Officer i/c Maternity Unit and "B" Block wards.

Miss Sinclair - Nursing Officer i/c "C" Block surgical wards and C.S.S.D. supplies.

Mr. Bastin - formerly Theatre Superintendent, appointed Nursing Officer i/c Casualty, O.P.D. and Theatres.

All three to be known as Unit Matrons.

At the end of 1970 the plans for the new intensive care/recovery unit had been agreed and work started on the building on 18th January, 1971.

The question of providing a playgroup or creche for the children of staff working in the hospital was being seriously investigated.

1971 Industrial Disputes

In January, 1971, the power workers' national industrial dispute took place. The hospital maintenance department worked wonders in keeping the hospital electrical supply going. Mr. Thurston of Burwell kindly loaned a portable generator which was a great help. This dispute made the Regional Engineer think and in April, 1972, a standby generator, which met all the hospital requirements was installed. This was part of a Regional scheme and met all the hospital needs in case of a power cut.

Also at this time the postal workers' national industrial dispute took place. When scratching about it was found all the large hospitals had transport of some sort already doing journeys to their respective Group HQ and a form of inter-Group transport already existed. The RHB had a transport service to and from the Ministry of Health and with some adjustments a very wide postal service between hospitals, Groups, Regions and the Ministry was set up. Patients were asked to telephone or call at the hospital and staff living in villages near the hospital were asked to act as postmen for the patients. The emergency system worked very well.

Miss Jenkins, the hospital Catering Officer, who had retired, was succeeded by Mr. E. H. Eyre from 15th March and Mr. A. J. Scotcher was appointed Voluntary Services Organiser on 16th March. This was a voluntary post and we were very lucky to obtain his services. Also in March a German-made meal vending machine was purchased and installed in the staff restaurant. It was available at any time during the day or night but its main purpose was to provide a better service for the night staff. A money change machine was installed a little later. The only other vending machine of its kind was in use at the Police HQ in Cambridge where it was seen working before we made the purchase.

In April the new Milton sterilizing unit was installed in the maternity unit.

Pressure to open a staff playgroup or creche was increasing and it was proposed this should be housed in the original labour ward in "A" Block, previously used as the consultant medical staff sitting room. The unit was opened shortly afterwards.

In 1971 there was again difficulty in housing staff. Technical and trained nursing staff were not available locally and had to be recruited from afar. The hospital had limited accommodation for single staff and the Urban District Council were very difficult and did not assist in housing and this added to the hospital recruitment problem. In March the Chairman of the HMC was asked to make an official request to the Council for an allocation of housing accommodation. There was some response to his request but the problem remained, although the Council kindly offered the use of 2 Challise Close, Saxon Street, the offer being gratefully accepted.

In June the Voluntary Organiser reported fifty-four voluntary workers were giving an average of 370 hours of voluntary work each week, mainly on the geriatric wards.

On 17th July a public meeting was held at the hospital and a Hospital League of Friends formed. Mr. H. Day was elected Chairman. The League has gone from strength to strength over the years and now plays an important part in the day to day life of the hospital.

At the July meeting of the House Committee it was reported with regret that Dr. Norman Gray and Captain H. R. King had died. They had both done excellent work for the hospital. Miss M. Hayward, the outpatient department sister and the sister in charge of Ward C9, retired in July after twenty-three years' service.

On 8th October the first Hospital Awards Day was held. This included the presentation of Awards to all hospital staff who had passed examinations. Mr. S. Alper, Chairman of Caravans International Ltd., presented the awards. In previous years the Annual Prizegiving had been confined to nursing staff.

It was reported in October that there were fifty pupil nurses in post: the establishment was increased to eighty-two.

Mr. Scotcher, the Voluntary Services Organiser, left on 12th October. Mrs. J. Amdrus was his successor on a full-time basis but the appointment was not successful.

In December the death of Mrs. O'Callaghan was reported. She had been a long standing member of the BRCS and a member of the Hospital House Committee.

In 1971 the staff health centre was opened. Dr. J. M. Platts was appointed staff health officer and introduced medical examinations for all hospital employees, not only for nursing staff, together with immunisation and access to the staff health centre for advice and investigation.

At this time there were so many hospital projects being put forward and it was difficult to decide on priorities. They were called the "Newmarket Jigsaw".

1972 New Day Hospital

The work on the new recovery/intensive care unit, attached to the theatres, was completed on 16th November, 1971 and in January, 1972, a work study commenced on the hospital medical records department. This was very necessary since requests for extra staff and equipment had been refused on grounds of cost. The necessary funds were, however, found following the work study.

Plans for a completely new day hospital in "B" Block had been agreed and Messrs. Kerridge Ltd. of Cambridge completed the construction work on 31st March. The new department was opened by Mr. G. S. Gibson, pictured here.

In May Sister Wedgewood, who had been the sister i/c Ward B6, was appointed sister in charge of the new day hospital.

© Cambridge Evening News

On 1st July the Newmarket Rotary Club sponsored a horse race meeting at the July course at Newmarket to raise funds for the hospital and on 17th July contractors work started on building an extension to the maternity unit to provide a new nursery and ancillary rooms. The work was completed in March, 1973.

On 7th August Mr. Cairns and Mr. Watson moved their ophthalmic unit to the new premises at Addenbrooke's Hospital and ward C5 was closed. The services of Sister Evans and the other Addenbrooke's nursing staff was withdrawn. I remember a very nice party was held in the ward on the final day. The ward had done excellent work and they were all missed very much.

In August a terrace house, 60 Exning Road, was purchased by the Ministry of Health. It accommodated nursing staff. On 4th December the Ministry agreed the purchase of 89 St. Phillips Road as a nurses' residence.

On 4th December a work study on the hospital catering service started.

The Chartered Society of Physiotherapists were given permission by the HMC to adapt the hospital physiotherapy film for national use. It was very much in demand.

Also in December Miss M. Armstrong, Senior Nursing Officer, resigned to take up a post with the Ministry of Health in London.

Cambridgeshire County Council provided a special ambulance to convey patients living in the Cambridgeshire villages to and from the day hospital. The arrangements made by the West Suffolk County Council left much to be desired.

1973

On 1st January, 1973, Mr. B. M. Witley, the Group Fire Officer, died suddenly. Mr. W. S. Green succeeded him, being appointed from 1st April.

Dr. Arden Jones' Rheumatoid Arthritis Research Project was concluded. It had been running since 1968. Also in January a forty-hour working week was introduced for all nursing staff. Authority was given to appoint a further four part-time ward clerks.

Miss D. Drake was appointed Deputy Medical Records Officer on 22nd May. She had worked in the administrative office since joining the hospital staff in 1940.

About this time the possibility of making a ring road round the hospital was being examined. The idea was to extend the "C" entrance road via the boiler house to the Field Terrace Road entrance. It would mean purchasing a small strip of land from the Hon. Mrs. Lambton and the scheme was not proceeded with. The possibility of using the County Library Service was also being looked into. It was agreed that our request would be considered after the service had been introduced in the new West Suffolk Hospital in Bury St. Edmunds.

In April the coronary care unit was opened in Ward B2. Part of the ward was partitioned off to form the unit. A purpose built, separate unit was wanted but funds did not allow. The normal ward staff ran the unit as part of their day to day work. There was also in April an ancillary staff industrial dispute. The staff restaurant was closed for some time making life very difficult. The hospital was not used to these actions and this had a very bad effect on the morale of all the staff.

In June, 1973, a series of lectures and classes were held for trained nursing staff and those interested in returning to nursing as a result of the "Back to Nursing Campaign". On 19th June the NHS Advisory Team (Geriatrics) visited the hospital to inspect the geriatric service which was building up into a comprehensive unit. They were very helpful and made a number of suggestions.

In June the original porters' lodge receiving rooms, etc. were demolished and the front of the hospital cleaned up. In July the hospital medical records department introduced a new system of patients mechanical documentation. This was part of the work study report.

The Editor of the Newmarket Journal reported that the Journal Christmas Fund had raised a record sum of £1,803 during 1973. This was the paper's centenary year and a number of special events had been held. We were very grateful.

1974 *Management Change Again*

In February, 1974, Dr. C. P. Hay and Mr. E. S. Jamieson retired. They had both been with the hospital for many years and their services were very much missed. It has already been said that Mr. Jamieson and Miss Welply had run the hospital accident department single-handedly almost since its opening and when they were no longer there, there was a shake-up of the accident and emergency services. Mr. D. Dandy, Consultant Orthopaedic Surgeon, succeeded Mr. Jamieson and he fought long and hard to put the service on a proper basis.

On 4th June Miss S. M. Stevens, Superintendent Physiotherapist retired. She was succeeded by Miss G. Hodge.

The Hospital House Committee, which had been in existence in one form or another since the original workhouse was built, was disbanded. The last meeting was held in March, 1974. The administration of the hospital had changed so much that the House Committee were no longer necessary. The NHS was reorganised again in April, 1974, and management was again changing.

Chapter Ten

THE FIRST REORGANISATION OF THE NATIONAL HEALTH SERVICE

April, 1974

On 1st April, 1974, the NHS was reorganised and this coincided with the reorganisation of Local Government. It was decided that the new Local Authorities should no longer be made responsible for any part of the health services and, with a few exceptions, all the health services for both primary and secondary care were brought together to form a unified health service. Administration was to be by line management, roughly speaking, that is a departmental officer at each tier of the structure, thus the catering department had a Regional, Area and District Catering Officer in each main hospital who supervised the day to day work of the department.

On paper the attraction of the scheme is obvious, in practice it proved extremely cumbersome to operate.

The East Anglian Regional Health Authority (RHA) was still based in Cambridge. The Suffolk Area Health Authority (AHA) was based in Ipswich and, again, the Region followed the county boundaries. The County of Suffolk was divided into the Ipswich Health District and the Bury St. Edmunds Health District and Newmarket General Hospital was part of this latter District. At this level there were District Management Teams (DMT) consisting of an Administrator, a Finance Officer, a Nursing Officer and a Community Physician, with a representative from the general practitioners and hospital consultant medical staff.

The internal management for the new service was set up in what came to be called the "Grey Book" in England and the "Red Book" in Wales ("Management Arrangements for the Reorganised National Health Service: HMSO 1972). The Hospital Secretary was renamed Unit Administrator and hardly knew where he was. One important change was that the hospital social work, always carried out by the almoner, was transferred to the Social Service department who worked on a county basis. They would only deal with problems of patients living in Suffolk. Eventually the needs of the patients living in Cambridgeshire were incorporated into one department with duplicate staff, for each county. Mrs. Bell had done this work, most satisfactorily, singlehanded for a very long time.

As the new service developed more and more departments were controlled on the line management basis from Area and this was confusing for the hospital staff. The pathology department added to this confusion by being put under the administrative control of the Cambridge Health District (Teaching). The department had always worked closely with Addenbrooke's Hospital and the Cambridge Public Health laboratories.

The Unit Administrator took over the day to day administration of the health clinics at Newmarket and Mildenhall and some other odds and ends such as staff houses. One of these was a radio aerial station near Chevely. We went to look at this and found it unmanned and locked up and, apparently, because it was a relay aerial for the ambulance service, as well as the police, etc. they thought Newmarket General Hospital should look after it. We didn't!

The 1970's were difficult years: the new system was being implemented, the trade unions were taking a much more active role and the conflicting interests of different professional groups were causing trouble. Towards the end of 1974 discussions on a new contract for consultant medical staff broke down and there were restrictions in services offered by consultants and specialists. For a period in 1975 junior doctors restricted their work to emergencies because of discontent over delays in introducing changes in their remuneration. The ancillary staff were also taking industrial action. However, bringing together the primary and secondary care was a good thing and, slowly, a more combined service came into being. The local clinics were able to make use of the hospital services and become involved with the hospital work.

The first meeting of the DMT at Bury St. Edmunds took place on 1st April, 1974. Mr. F. R. Rich, the District Administrator, was made Chairman. Mr. P. M. Cooke, the former Group Secretary, had been promoted to the post of Area Administrator at Ipswich.

On 20th April a report on a proposed Area Staff Consultative Scheme was being considered. These staff consultative meetings had previously been held locally and local action taken.

The Accident and Emergency service at Newmarket General Hospital was under review and meetings were held at the hospital with local general practitioners to discuss the position and see if their services could be used in any way.

Dr. N. Coni, Consultant Geriatrician, requested water beds for use on the geriatric wards. In the old days these were always used and fortunately there were two still in store.

By April an Area Training Officer, based in Ipswich, had been appointed. The requirements of the Fire Precautions Act 1971 were being considered. When implemented a certificate for the hospital premises would be issued. The Hospital Secretary had always been the hospital fire officer but under the stricter new rules it was difficult to make any one officer responsible since the hospital is open twenty-four hours a day the year round.

In June there was a shortage of beds for diseases of the chest and Dr. C. Lum, Consultant Chest Physician, requested a new chest unit be provided. The hospital was also being pressed to operate a psychiatric service but there were no beds available at the time for either specialty.

In July there was unrest again amongst the members of COHSE and NUPE, as well as amongst the members of NALGO representing radiographers and engineers. In August a contractors' specialised cleaning service was introduced into the hospital kitchen.

In the autumn of 1974 the new "Best Buy" West Suffolk Hospital was opened in Bury St. Edmunds. When first opened it had very little effect on the work of Newmarket General Hospital.

1975 *Pathology Transfer*

On 5th February, 1975, the administrative control of the pathology department was transferred to the Cambridge Health District (Teaching) based at Addenbrooke's Hospital.

At this time the morale of the ancillary staff was very low. The domestic staff went on strike on 1st March: they were supported by the catering staff. This was over the bonus scheme introduced by the work study team and a new bonus scheme for the domestic staff. The DMT approved expenditure of £26,670.

On 5th March the DMT recommended that the accident and emergency department be closed. This was being considered by the AHA and a public meeting was held in the Memorial Hall, Newmarket. Mr. H. Day was the Chairman and Dr. G. Patey, the District Community Physician, acted as spokesman.

On 23rd April the provision of a new post graduate medical centre in "C" Block was approved at a cost of £15,000.

In June it was reported that the patients' pillow radio service had come to the end of its useful life. A new four channel system was required. The Hospital League of Friends donated £1,000 and the DMT made a further £1,000 available for half the new system to be provided. In June, too, the ambulance men notified they were taking industrial action.

In July the domestic staff firmly rejected the proposed bonus scheme. The approved expenditure of £26,670 was reconsidered. Following a report by Mr. J. S. Knox, the District Domestic Manager, it was agreed that one extra supervisor and six extra domestic workers be employed at a cost of £14,169. It was some time before the bonus scheme was agreed.

In September the RHA instructed that no further incentive bonus schemes were to be implemented. In October the Area scheme of the Joint Staff Consultative Committee was brought into being. The direct link between the hospital and the DMT was to remain. A member of the hospital JSCC would act as representative on the Area Council and staff consultation took on a much wider basis.

Also in October, the future role of Newmarket General Hospital was being considered again. The Cambridge AHA said they would be requiring the same amount of service from the hospital for the foreseeable future.

In November the junior medical staff at the West Suffolk Hospital and at Newmarket General Hospital took industrial action over the new proposed medical staff contracts. Later they were supported by the senior medical staff.

During the same month 23 Field Terrace Road and 60 Exning Road were sold with a view to purchasing more suitable accommodation. In the following month, the hospital residential accommodation was again giving trouble. It was considered well below the standard required. A plan to build an eighty unit purpose built block was being considered.

An application was made to convert the old laundry building into a small indoor swimming pool. Mr. G. Gibson gave valuable advice on the day to day running of such a pool. The cost then was £16,000 and the annual running costs would be at least £2,500. A visit to the Forest Health District Council at Mildenhall revealed that the Council intended to build a new swimming pool for the town close to the hospital on the new George Lambton estate. The hospital scheme was dropped and, apparently, so was the District Council scheme. This was unfortunate.

1976 Low Morale

In January, 1976, Mr. W. S. Green, who had been the Group Fire Officer, based at Newmarket General Hospital, was appointed District Fire Officer and his office moved to the old St. Mary's Hospital site at Bury St. Edmunds.

On 15th January a meeting with hospital staff and the local general practitioners was held at the hospital to consider restricted hours of opening of the accident and emergency department. It was agreed, with immediate effect, that the hours the department would be open in future would be from 9 a.m. to 5.30 p.m. daily, Monday to Friday.

On 16th and 17th March the Medicines Inspectors visited the hospital pharmacy. They were considering the suitability of the premises and equipment for carrying out activities listed for a manufacturing licence. The RHA had agreed the department being extended to supply the Area needs.

In March the ambulance service staff again took industrial action. This had a bad effect on outpatient clinics. In April the C.S.S.D. sterilised pack system was started in the accident and casualty department. This service was extended to the local general practitioners' surgeries on a weekly top-up basis.

In May the RHA were concerned about the number of accidents to staff in preparing topical water. Glass containers were used for the water and when sterilizing was complete and the sterilizer doors opened the cold air met the hot glass containers and some often exploded injuring the staff. A scheme to centralize the sterilizing at Bury St. Edmunds had been prepared. Newmarket General Hospital had been a centre for supplying this topical water, not only to theatre and maternity, but also to other hospitals in the old Group. The large old American steriliser in "C" Block was ideal for the purpose and the Head Porter was instructed to do the sterilizing at 4 p.m. each day and when complete to lock the sterilizing room door. It would be opened the following morning when all the glass bottles were cold and no more accidents occurred. However, the new unit was opened at Bury St. Edmunds and the high cost of providing the new service was giving considerable concern.

In the spring of 1976 Dr. Arden Jones retired after giving thirty-six years of invaluable service to the hospital.

In May the building work for the new post graduate medical educational centre and the upgrading of the adjoining staff recreation room was underway. Mr.

G. Gibson had helped, financially, with the improvements to the staff recreation room and it was decided to call the unit the Gibson Centre.

In June schemes were being prepared as follows:

Improved office accommodation for social workers	£ 4,600
Extension of sanitary annex between Wards B3 and B5 (geriatric)	£ 22,000
Improvements to X-ray department including a third diagnostic room	£115,000

It was quite some time before the plans for the X-ray department were agreed.

Dr. S. Ellis had been appointed Area Pharmaceutical Officer and the Inspectors' report on the hospital pharmacy was being considered. It was the intention of the RHA to centralise the pharmacy services at Newmarket and the Inspectors' report and the appointment of a senior member of the pharmacy staff was to this end. The scheme did not materialise: the service was centralised under the control of the Area Pharmacist at Ipswich.

In July there was a lot of local concern that the hospital accident and emergency department might close. An extra surgical registrar post was required to keep the service going but the Department of Health (DoH) would not agree to this. The East Cambridge District Council wrote to the DoH stating that in their view it was essential for the department to be kept open on the present basis. Mr. Eldon Griffiths, MP for Bury St. Edmunds and Newmarket, was concerned and chaired a meeting at the hospital with the staff of Newmarket and West Suffolk Hospitals and other people concerned.

The Hospital Activity Analysis for 1975 for Cambridge showed that sixty per cent of the geriatric patients admitted to Newmarket General Hospital came from the Cambridge Health District.

The junior medical staff had taken industrial action in February and again in July over the conditions of their new contracts. The terms were finally agreed in September and everyone was very relieved.

In December the morale of the telephonists was low: the trade unions were involved.

1977 Dick Heasman Retires

In January, 1977, the low bed occupancy for dental, general practitioner maternity, obstetrics and gynaecology was noted and a better use of these beds was sought from the medical staff.

In February the second and final phase of upgrading the staff recreation room (Gibson Centre) was started and Mr. M. Bright, Consultant Obstetrician & Gynaecologist, submitted a plan to the DMT for new labour wards and admission block to be built alongside the maternity unit in "A" Block. The plan was agreed in principle.

On 16th March the Thursday morning ante-natal session held at Newmarket General Hospital was moved to Mildenhall Health Centre. It was changed to Wednesday afternoons since there was very limited public transport from Mildenhall to Newmarket.

On 26th April Dr. G.M.W. Kerrigan and Dr. I. Evans, Consultant Physicians, submitted a case to the DMT for the provision of a full and adequate coronary care unit at Newmarket.

Mr. R. W. Heasman, Unit Administrator, retired on 14th May, 1977 being succeeded from 31st August by Mr. G. Newbury.

The planned alterations to the X-ray department had been prepared by Dr. J. P. Williams and when Dr. Hatcher was appointed as Consultant Radiologist to succeed him the proposed alterations were reviewed and updated. This involved extending the department to provide one extra diagnostic room and became a major capital development at an estimated cost of £350,000.

The telephonists were still giving trouble. Full meetings were held between management and all the unions.

In July the psychiatric service was still difficult. The whole of Suffolk, including Newmarket, still came under St. Audrey's Hospital, Ipswich. It was stressed that there was an urgent need for a proper psychiatric service in the Newmarket and Haverhill areas.

In November the long term role of Newmarket General Hospital was again under discussion by the DMT.

On 16th December an aeroplane from the American base at Lakenheath crashed in a field on Scaltback estate which is close to the hospital. Fortunately there were no casualties but another look was taken at the Major Accident Plan. It was considered that a full exercise between the Health Districts should be held every three years and any local schemes should be checked.

The contract for the nurses' assisted travel scheme was put out to tender and Messrs. Youngs Coaches was given the contract for the Cambridge run and Messrs. Miller Bros. Ltd. the Haverhill run.

1978 *Regional Centre for Rheumatology*

In March, 1978, the future use of the facilities at Newmarket General Hospital were again under discussion, particularly in view of the estimated limited life of the buildings and the requirements of Cambridge, in view of the opening of the new Hinchingbrooke Hospital in Huntingdon. It was suggested that both Districts would benefit if they worked together with mutual advantage towards better and more extensive use of resources at Newmarket.

In June the hospital telephone exchange was moved to much better accommodation in "A" Block and the staff were much happier.

Handicapped children from the Roger Ascham School were using the hydrotherapy pool.

Following a linen count £5,000 was allocated to meet one year's losses of standard items of linen.

On 20th June the final plans for the conversion of Wards B4 and B6 were agreed. Dr. C. Lum stressed the future needs for additional chest beds and in October the Medical Staff Committee recommended that Ward C5 should be used as a Rheumatology Unit. This was the start of the development of a Regional Centre for Rheumatology at Newmarket.

1979 *Industrial Action Again*

On 22nd January, 1979, the ancillary staff and some nursing staff in the District took industrial action in their campaign against low pay. NUPE and COHSE trade unions were involved. An emergency control committee was set up at each hospital and a National Code of Practice for emergency services had been agreed with the trade unions. Admissions ceased. On 23rd February agreement with the trade unions was reached and normal admissions resumed. They were difficult times.

In March the RHA agreed the plans to upgrade the geriatric Wards B4 and B6 and to the extension of the scheme to meet the needs of the patients with diseases of the chest which Dr. Lum had been pressing for.

In April concern was again expressed over the lack of service for psychogeriatric patients in the Newmarket and Haverhill areas. Complaints were again being received from relatives living in the Haverhill area that members of their family were still being sent to St. Audrey's Hospital near Ipswich. The Cambridgeshire AHA proposed a revision of the sectorisation of the area covered by Fulbourn Hospital to cover Newmarket and Haverhill. Unfortunately, there was no progress.

Provisional approval was given to the expenditure of £110,000 on equipment and other items for the new Regional Rheumatology Centre at Newmarket General Hospital.

During April Mr. D. J. Dandy, Consultant Orthopaedic Surgeon, was made Hon. Secretary of the District Medical Committee for the integration of the orthopaedic departments at Addenbrooke's and Newmarket Hospitals.

In June the scheme for the new labour suite attached to the maternity department and also for the maintenance staffs' new workshops attached to the boiler house in "C" Block, were submitted to the RHA for consideration.

In September a scheme had been put forward to use Ward A3 in "A" Block for gynaecology day surgery cases. The cost of this was £56,000 and the scheme was deferred in view of the reallocation of surgical beds and the development of the Regional Centre for Rheumatology.

In July the Bury St. Edmunds Health District were concerned about the cross-boundary flow of funds in relation to patients living in Cambridgeshire being admitted to Newmarket General Hospital. That dreadful County boundary has always been a nightmare to the work of Newmarket General Hospital.

The AHA required vigorous attention to be given to the conservation of energy. The DMT stipulated that the temperatures in all areas be reduced from 71 to 68 degrees. This was left open for discussion and I am not sure if it was implemented. In August a report on hygiene was received from the District

Catering Manager. This was made following a planned inspection of all hospitals in the District by the DoH Inspectors.

In September the introduction of microfilming of patients' medical records, at a cost of £3,500, was agreed in principle.

By October the RHA had approved the development of the Regional Rheumatology Unit at Newmarket General Hospital and set the target date for completion as 1st April, 1980.

In December it was agreed that the wiring of the patients' radio system should be renewed. "C" Block was renewed first at a cost of £4,000, the cost being met from Hospital Free Monies, Mr. Gibson's Trust Fund and the Newmarket Journal Christmas Fund.

The DMT agreed the operational policy of the physiotherapy department should incorporate provision for open access to the department by general practitioners, who could refer patients direct to the department without going through outpatient clinics.

1980 *Accident Unit Closed*

In January, 1980, it was learned that it was proposed to reduce the number of diseases of the chest beds at Papworth Hospital and there was concern as to how this would effect the beds at Newmarket. This helped Dr. Lum's case for more beds.

The DMT agreed to provide funds for Ward C3 to open as a female surgical ward run on a seven day basis. Mr. Graham Jones, prospective Liberal Candidate, held a public meeting in the Newmarket Library on 31st January to discuss the future of this ward. The ward was opened in March the designation being changed from children's ward to female surgical ward. Ward C5 was also opened in March as a Rheumatology Unit. The official opening ceremony was performed by Professor John Butterfield, OBE, MD, FRCP, Regius Professor of Physic at Cambridge University, on 31st October. Mr. J. T. Dingle, D.Sc., Ph.D., Director of Strangeways Research Laboratory in Cambridge, was also a guest speaker.

Dr. J. H. Dean, Consultant Pathologist, retired on 1st June, 1980, although he worked as a locum on several occasions thereafter.

On 4th August the male geriatric/chest ward was temporarily closed to allow the contractors' work on upgrading Wards B4 and B6. The ward remained closed until the new year.

In September the DoH proposed to change direction in its policy of hospital services with less concentration of beds in the large District General Hospitals, with consequent greater use of existing local hospitals. The estimated geographical population needs for 1991 were noted and also that the Bury St. Edmunds District had the largest growth rate in the Region. The DMT were opposed to any reduction in the beds at the West Suffolk Hospital, Bury St. Edmunds. The maximum proposed beds were 677.

In September Dr. Hatcher reported to the DMT that Messrs. AgfaGevaert, agents, wished to introduce logetronic equipment into this country and the equipment would be made available, free of charge, during the trial period at Newmarket General Hospital. This was agreed for a six month period: Dr. Hatcher to have the assistance of the Department of Physics at Addenbrooke's Hospital, Cambridge.

Mr. Fred Rich, the District Administrator, retired on 31st October, 1980.

In November it was reported that the accident and emergency department at Newmarket had closed. On two occasions the department had been referred to as a minor accident and emergency department. Usually these are run by the local general practitioners and exist in many towns like Sudbury, Thetford, Southwold, etc. It is a shame that when the main accident department was closed such a unit was not left in its place. Newmarket town is developing at a very fast rate.

In December a request was received from the Dean of the Clinical School at Cambridge for the placement of additional medical students at Newmarket General Hospital for training in general medicine, chest medicine, gastroenterology and rheumatology from May to October, 1981. Accommodation was difficult.

1981 *Awaiting Another Reorganisation*

In January, 1981, the possibility of mounting a Joint Board of Clinical Nursing Studies in Rheumatology course at Newmarket General Hospital was being investigated.

The official opening of the new X-ray Department took place on 30th April when the guest of honour was Miss A. Cowper-Johnson, a former long-serving Superintendent Radiographer.

On 1st June the local general practitioners were given open access to the occupational therapy department in the same manner as enjoyed in the physiotherapy department. The patients requiring standard treatments could be referred direct without having to attend the consultant outpatient clinic. This was done for a six month period at the end of which it was found the demand was relatively small and the service continued on a permanent basis.

In July it was reported that the work of the ambulance stations at Newmarket and Mildenhall had been monitored since the closure of the hospital accident and emergency department. The service provided was well within the national norm and the closure of the department had not had any effect on the level of service provided for the town and surrounding villages.

In November the DMT felt they could not recommend funding the following capital developments until such time as the future development policy of the hospital had been clearly determined:

(a) relocation of the cardiac unit in Ward B2.
(b) improved sanitary facilities in Wards C6-C7. C8-C9, B1-B2.
(c) improvements to the operating theatre changing facilities.

Chapter Eleven

THE RESTRUCTURED NATIONAL HEALTH SERVICE 1982

As mentioned earlier, the Health Service was again restructured in 1982. The Area Health Authorities (AHA) were removed and District Health Authorities (DHA) introduced with General Managers at both the District and Hospital levels. The new structure was much closer to the hospitals and the patients and the Hospital General Manager was given much more authority. The Bury St. Edmunds Health District became the West Suffolk Health Authority. The Department of Health and Social Security (DHSS) requested views on determining boundaries of the new DHAs in the new NHS reorganisation.

On 4th January, 1982, a case of salmonella infection was found in Ward B3. All precautions were taken and the ward was closed for a short time.

In March the RHA made application to the DHSS for the designation of Newmarket General Hospital as a Demonstration Centre in Medical Rehabilitation (Rheumatology). This was agreed on 13th April. In March, too, a new electrocardiograph machine was purchased at a cost of £3,600. The cost was shared between the Hospital Free Monies account and the Hospital League of Friends.

In April Dr. J. M. Platts retired after forty years service with the hospital. She and Mr. E. S. Heasman, who was the original Workhouse Master and later Clerk and Steward, were the longest serving members of staff. Others were:

Mr. E. S. Heasman	40 years
Dr. J. M. Platts	40 years
Mr. R. W. Heasman	37 years
Miss D. Drake	36 years
Mr. J. S. Garmory	34 years
Mrs. D. Parr	29 years

Miss A. Penne, Senior Nursing Officer until 1st September, 1980, then acting Divisional Nursing Officer, retired in November, 1982. She was awarded the MBE for her many years of excellent nursing service.

In October a meeting between the new West Suffolk and Cambridge DMTs was held at the hospital to discuss the Newmarket development proposals. The strategies outlined in the document envisaged a continuing role for Newmarket General Hospital both complementing the provision of acute specialties in the West Suffolk Hospital and continuing to serve that part of East Cambridgeshire which had always looked to Newmarket for hospital services.

The staffing situation at Newmarket was still one of the key issues in the redevelopment. It was considered necessary to totally rebuild the hospital because of its poor structural condition. It was also necessary for the long term strategy to be clearly set out.

1983 Complete Rebuilding Plans

In January, 1983, the Newmarket Unit Management Group (UMG) was formed. This was based on a report from Mr. J. R. Melleney, the newly-appointed District Administrator of the newly-formed West Suffolk Health Authority, which set up five managerial units in West Suffolk, viz West Suffolk and Thetford, Newmarket, Community Services, Sudbury and Mental Handicap Services. This followed the thrust of Circular HC(80)8 of July 1980 to provide maximum delegation to units for decision making at that unit level, within policies laid down by the Health Authority and the DMT acting on its behalf. The UMG met on 7th April with the following members present:

Mr. G. Newbury	Unit Administrator.
Miss L. E. Bowyer	Director of Nursing Services
Mr. M. V. Bright	Chairman, Medical Staff Committee
Dr. G. N. W. Kerrigan	Secretary, Medical Staff Committee
Mr. N. Robinson	Unit Management Accountant.

On 12th May a request was received from the University of Cambridge Clinical School to provide support for a new post of University Lecturer in Orthopaedics to undertake three consultant sessions at Newmarket General Hospital - one surgical list, one outpatient clinic and one ward round. The West Suffolk DMT agreed.

In June the furniture in the Board Room was sold. This was rather a shame since it had been in place since the original Workhouse was built. Also in June a report on the work of the chest unit was received, which showed an expansion of outpatient attendances from 170 to 350 and the annual number of inpatients rising from 130 to 340.

In June Miss E. J. Harvey was appointed Superintendent Physiotherapist and Mrs. J. Haslam, Hospital Medical Records Officer. Mr. R. E. B. Tagart, Consultant General Surgeon, retired in August.

We all look, with interest, to see how the restructured NHS with the increasing amount of private medicine meets the needs of the British people. From this history alone, one can see the British have more experience of a NHS than any other country. Let's hope, this time, we shall get the best service possible for the money we provide.

The decision to completely rebuild Newmarket General Hospital was taken in 1982 and I feel this is an appropriate time for me to conclude this history. The original buildings in "A" Block were built about 150 years ago and have been altered and extended so many times over the years. "B" and "C" Block buildings were built in the early years of the second world war and, like the prefabs, were only intended to last for ten years. Whatever materials were available locally were used and these were in very short supply. The standard of the buildings in "B" Block was poor for this reason.

The hospital, as it stands, has served the people in the district well and we all look forward to the arrival of the new buildings.

The excellent work goes on and this is borne out by the wonderful support the hospital continues to receive from the local people. Its good reputation was built, over the years, on the work of many dedicated members of staff and, unfortunately, only a few can be mentioned in this history. Let's hope the younger generation will continue to strive for improvements and, sometimes, give a thought to the good work, through difficult times, of their predecessors.

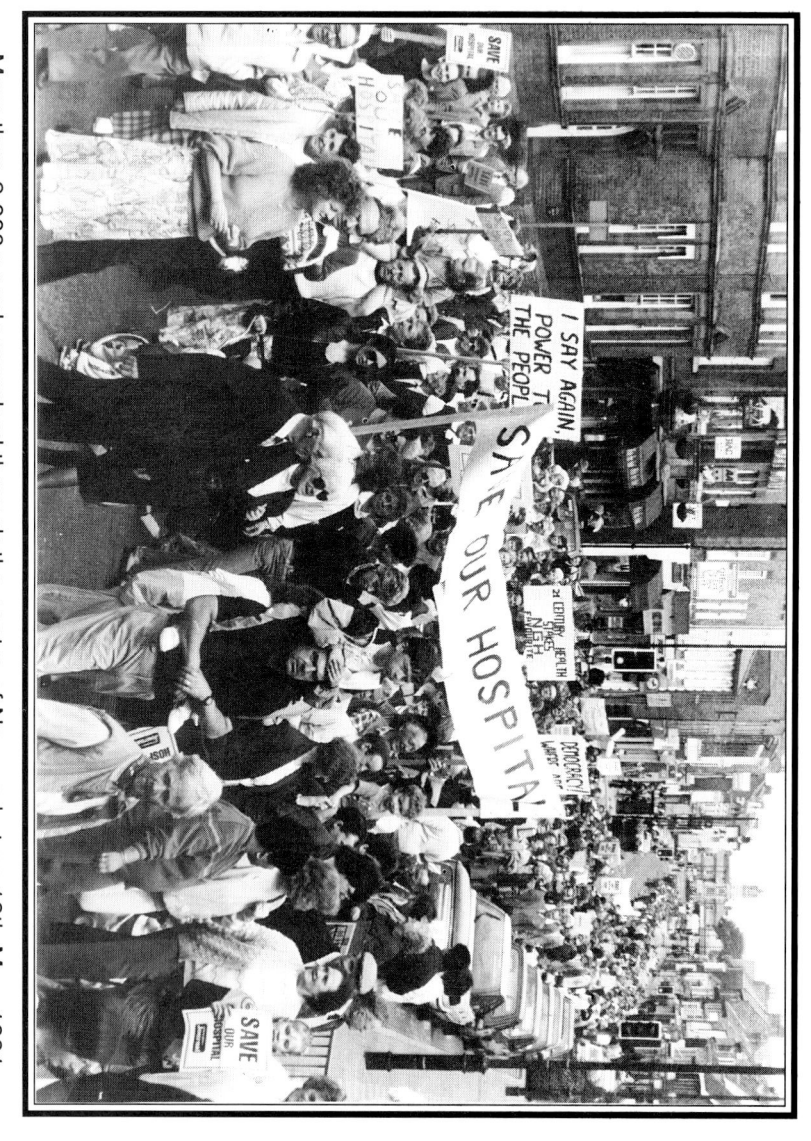

More than 9,000 people marched through the centre of Newmarket on 19th May, 1991, to protest at health authority plans to downgrade the hospital.

Photograph reproduced with kind permission of the East Anglian Daily Times.

148

Chapter Twelve

THE TROUBLED DECADE

1982 *New Health Authority*

It was noted with pleasure that from early February, 1982, two part-time phlebotomists had been appointed for out-patient work and that it was hoped inpatient work could be similarly covered in future.

The Hospital Medical Staff Committee (MSC) agreed to arrange a cocktail party at the hospital on 11th March to entertain, meet and welcome the new members appointed to serve on the West Suffolk Health Authority (WSHA), to be formed officially from 1st April.

On 6th April Dr. Brian Hazleman reported that the DHSS had designated the Hospital as a Demonstration Centre in Rheumatology: Newmarket General Hospital was one of twelve hospitals in the country so recognised.

Sister Wedgwood (Sister Day Centre) retired on 1st August and was replaced by Sister Claydon.

For information, a meeting of senior staff on 16th December, 1982, was well attended by the following staff representatives:

Miss S. Blakey	Dietitian
Mr. H. Mason	Head Gardener
Mr. F. Watts	Senior Chief MLSO
Miss A. Saunders	Staff Pharmacist
Mrs. Midgley-Revett	Medical Records Officer
Sister V. Skipp	Administrative Sister
Miss G. Hodge	Supt. Physiotherapist
Mr. E. Eyre	Catering Manager
Mrs. S. Hardy	Assistant Domestic Manager
Mrs. M. Bentinck	Linen Room Supervisor
Miss L. E. Bowyer	Director of Nursing Services
Mrs. E. Lee	Supt. Radiographer
Mr. A. K. North	Deputy Administrator

and the meeting was chaired by Mr. G. Newbery, the Administrator. For the complete record of senior staff, the following were unable to attend that meeting:

Miss A. Jones	Nursing Officer, Maternity
Miss M. Sinclair	Nursing Officer, C Block
Miss A. Lyimo	Nursing Officer, Theatre
Mrs. O. Jacobs	Nursing Officer, B. Block
Mrs. I. Bell	Medical Social Worker

1983 Unit Management Group

Everyone was delighted when Miss A. Penney, former Senior Nursing Officer, was awarded the MBE in the Honours Lists.

Based on a report from the District General Manager, which after discussion with senior staff, wide consultation and approval by the Health Authority, the Newmarket Unit Management Group was set up and had its first meeting on 7th April. Five managerial units were provided in the WSHA area, viz West Suffolk and Thetford, Newmarket, Community, Sudbury and Mental Handicap services. The philosophy was based on the thrust of circular HC(80)8 of July 1980 which aimed to provide maximum delegation to units for decision making at that level, within policies laid down by the HA and by DMT acting on its behalf. UMG members, by consensus decision, would have collective responsibility for deciding how resources were to be used and advising on development priorities.

It had been agreed that the UMG would comprise the Unit Administrator, the Director of Nursing Services and elected or nominated representatives of the medical staff. The UMG had powers to co-opt as necessary and were encouraged to have a treasurer to attend meetings on a regular basis. Minutes of all meetings would be published.

The first meeting on 7th April was attended by Mr. G Newbury, Miss L. E . Bowyer, Mr. M.V. Bright (Chairman MSC), Dr. G.N.W. Kerrigan (Secretary MSC) and Mr. N. Robinson as appointed Unit management accountant. The UMG planned to meet weekly thereafter.

Mr. R. Tagart gave notice that he planned to retire in July 1984. It was noted that Mr. Monkton was to retire in September 1983 and Mr. Robert Lamb was appointed to succeed him early in 1984.

Mr. D. Dandy was appointed Honorary Consultant in Orthopaedics to the Royal Navy and RAF in July.

In July the Regional Specialties and Services Working Party supported an application from Dr. J. Shneerson, Consultant Physician, for funding to establish a regional Assisted Ventilation Unit (AVU). This scheme had the support of the Hospital Medical Staff Committee, the West Suffolk Health Authority and the East Anglian Thoracic Medicine Advisory Committee.

The proposal was accepted in September and £16,000 was allocated for the construction of the unit, together with £10,500 per annum for five years to enable all the necessary equipment needed to provide patient care. The building work in Ward B4 was completed in 1984, providing seven bed spaces including two for tank ventilation (iron lung) care. The unit was officially opened by HRH Princess of Wales, Patron of the British Lung Foundation, in June 1988.

Sister Jean Berrigan was senior nurse sister on the ward from 1982 until 1984 and was succeeded by Sister V. McLeod, who stayed with the ward when its services were transferred to Papworth Hospital in February, 1992.

In later years Dr. Shneerson reported on remarkable clinical success and although the service was intended for the whole of East Anglia an increasing number of patients were referred from places as far away as Bournemouth, Exeter, Liverpool, Dundee and Aberdeen. It was acknowledged that the survival figures for patients were nearly 90% after one year of treatment and 85% after two years.

Miss E. Harvey was appointed Superintendent Physiotherapist, succeeding Miss G. Hodge, Mrs. J. Haslam as Medical Records Officer and Mr. B. Johnson as deputy administrator, succeeding Mr. A. K. North.

Hospital medical staff were disappointed to learn in August that the RHA had decided to provide an elective orthopaedic unit for the SW quadrant of the region at Hinchingbrooke Hospital in Huntingdon, rather than at Newmarket.

On 28th September the new works department, referred to on several occasions in the earlier text, was completed and formally opened by Mr. F. J. Rich, the former Group Secretary/District Administrator. It is sad to report that after all the years of waiting the building only lasted thirteen years, being demolished in 1995 to make way for the new hospital.

Dr. L. Culank, Consultant Pathologist expressed concern in November that the need for two outstanding inpatient phlebotomists had still not been met. The records of increased in-patient phlebotomy were examined.

Mr. G. Newbery resigned his post following a promotion to the post of Administrator to St. Albans City Hospital and left on 30th November. Arrangements were made for Mr. B. A. Burton, DHQ general administrator to attend UMG meetings for three months before Mr. E. Bull took up his post.

The new Labour suite in the Maternity department came into operation on 22nd November and was formally opened on 30th March, 1984, by Mrs. Elizabeth Sayers, Deputy Editor, Newmarket Journal.

The UMG supported an innovative suggestion by Mrs. J. Fairbairn, Head Occupational Therapist, to pay the training costs of an aide who was considered capable of undergoing formal occupational therapy training and qualification. It was agreed to meet half of the cost from free monies, the remainder to come from the occupational therapy department budget.

For reference purposes, the Consultant staff providing the in- and out-patient clinical services were at this time as follows:

Anaesthetics	Dr. B. R. Stead, Dr. A. J. Pearce, Dr. C. P. Watsham, Dr. E. A. Maher, Dr. van den Brul.
Dermatology	Dr. R. J. Pye.
E. N. T.	Mr. D. Moffat.
Geriatrics	Dr. N. K. Coni.
Gynaecology/Obstetrics	Mr. M. V. Bright, Miss M. M. R. Martin.
Medicine	Dr. G. N. W. Kerrigan, Dr. P. Siklos.
Neurology	Dr. I. M. W. Wilkinson.
Ophthalmology	Mr. R. Lamb.
Oral Surgery	Mr. E. W. B. Varley.
Orthopaedic Surgery	Mr. D. J. Dandy, Mr. P. M. Scott, Mr. N. Rushton.
Paediatrics	Dr. N. Roberton.
Pathology	Dr. L. Culank, Dr. M. Seaman, Dr. R. Warren, Dr. P. Cooper.
Radiology	Dr. L. Hatcher, Dr. G. Woods, Dr. Y. Steel.
Rheumatology	Dr. B. L. Hazleman, Dr. R. Jubb.
General Surgery	Mr. R. E. B. Tagart, Mr. M. McBrien, Prof. R. Y. Calne, Mr. K. Rolles.
Thoracic Medicine	Dr. J. Shneerson.

1984 New Senior Staff

The Nurses' Award evening was held on 9th February, 1984, when Dr. D. Bratherton, Consultant Radiotherapist was the guest of honour.

It was regretted that Home Place Convalescent Home closed on 29th February since many patients had been sent there in the past for convalescence after general and gynaecology surgery.

Mr. E. C. Bull was appointed Unit Administrator and attended his first UMG meeting on 23rd February. Miss A. Saunders, Staff Pharmacist left in April to be married in May, being replaced by Mrs. Purser from 4th June. Staff Nurse Haigh was appointed Sister for Ward C5.

The Newmarket Journal fund raised over £2,800 and was used to purchase an automatic lung ventilator for the operating theatre. The recurring problem of recruitment of ODAs was having an effect on theatre lists and attempts were made to recruit agency staff.

It was reported on 1st May that Mr. R.E.B. Tagart had been awarded a Huntarian Professorship: his medical colleagues congratulated him then and in June 1985 after his Huntarian oration.

The English National Board representative visited to inspect facilities for pupil nurse training on 26th and 27th July.

The League of Friends fete held in the hospital grounds on 9th June, was well attended and raised a record £3,900.

In July work started on Ward B4 to provide accommodation for the Assisted Ventilation Unit, under the care of Dr. J. Shneerson. The alteration and upgrading work was let on a 13 week contract and would provide an extra seven beds.

The area formed by the admin. block, "A" and "B" Nurses' Homes and the Blue room became a listed building in August 1984.

Mrs. Clare Purser was appointed Pharmacist and Miss A. R. van Woerden appointed Director of Midwifery Services for the whole District. Dr. Al Rafaie was appointed Consultant Pathologist to succeed Dr. J. H. Dean. Miss Bowyer, Director of Nursing Services, retired on 12th November after 26 years service.

Miss A. Dunachie was appointed to succeed her from 1st November, having worked at Newmarket Hospital some years earlier.

By way of light relief, in December the UMG thought there was some advantage in using synthetic Xmas trees in the wards, particularly since there was no fire risk or needle shedding. The Medical Staff Committee were informed and "....deplored the substitution of synthetic for organic trees, but accepted the need for this change."

Much discussion took place on Circular HC(83)14 - the Griffiths Report: but more of that later.

Mrs. J. Parton, was appointed Nursing Officer for Midwifery services.

1985 *Another Reorganisation*

Circular HC(83)14 became a hot potato and a live issue! A consultative paper was once again produced by the District General Manager on 25th April, 1985 on revised management arrangements. In it he proposed three units of general management (rather than five created on 1st April, 1983), viz West Suffolk, Thetford and Sudbury Hospitals, Newmarket, and Community and Mental Handicap, with a Unit General Manager for each with individual responsibility and accountability to the DGM for the managerial performances of the unit and, as a member of a District Management Board, involvement in and commitment to the decisions of the Board and WSHA.

In July, after a competitive tendering exercise involving domestic, catering and laundry services for all the District hospitals, the domestic service contract for Newmarket Hospital was let with Sunlight Hospital Services. Mrs. Sheila Hardy, who was the Hospital Assistant Domestic Services Manager, was appointed by Sunlight Services as their Location Manager. Detailed personnel discussions took place with all the domestic staff and some retired, some took redundancy and some were employed by Sunlight Services. A farewell party was held on Friday, 27th September for all domestic staff.

Dr. Hatcher retired on 31st May 1986. Dr. R . Bannon was appointed Consultant Radiologist at West Suffolk Hospital with two sessions at Newmarket. Dr. Adrian Crisp was appointed Consultant Rheumatologist, to work with Dr. Brian Hazleman, from 1st March.

An episode of the popular TV series "Lovejoy" was filmed at Newmarket

General Hospital on 30th October: A fee of £150 was paid into free monies for patient amenities.

Mr. E. Bull presented his suggested Unit management structure to the team, proposing that the UMG would consist of the Unit General Manager, Director of Nursing Services, Manager of Personnel and Support Services, a Unit Medical Representative and the Hon. Secretary of the MSC. The UMG discussed future management arrangements and agreed that in future the UMG should also include the Unit Management Accountant. It was agreed that the Unit General Manager would discuss these management arrangements with the Medical Staff Committee (MSC).

At the first meeting in April Mr. D. J. Dandy (Unit Medical Representative), Dr. J. Shneerson (Hon. Secretary, MSC), Mr. B. Johnson (Manager of Personnel & Support Services) and Mr.N. Robinson (Unit Management Accountant) joined Mr. Bull and Miss Dunachie to form the UMG.

On 10th January, 1986, it was reported that upgrading work on Ward B1 would start on 4th February and in June it was announced, with great pleasure, that Mr. Leo Maycock, Senior Operating Department Assistant, had been awarded the B.E.M. in the Queen's Birthday Honours List. The Award was presented by the Lord Lieutenant of Suffolk, Sir Joshua Rowley, in the Gibson Centre on Wednesday, 8th October when many of Leo's relatives and many friends and colleagues were able to be present.

The Unit Management Group, which had been in existence since 1985, changed its title to Senior Management Group and agreed to meet weekly at 8.15 a.m. so that its clinical members could attend before their clinical duties. The membership remained as before, although Miss Dunachie's title changed in July to Nursing & Patient Care Manager.

Whilst there was continuing difficulty with the recruitment of ODA and theatre porters, it was pleasing to note that Mr. Colin Kennedy, recently appointed Consultant Urologist for West Suffolk and Newmarket Hospitals, was in a position to take up his outpatient and theatre sessions at Newmarket.

In August it was noted that £4,200 needed to be spent on upgrading the signposting throughout the hospital to comply with current regulations and with the views of the Hospital Advisory Team, who had visited the hospital.

On 18th October an Open Day in the Pathology Laboratory block took place to allow members of the public an opportunity to see the range of work carried out and Dr. Roger Pulvertaft took up his post of Consultant Radiologist, replacing Dr. Hatcher. In the same month Ward C7 was closed temporarily, reopening as a four day ward, from Tuesday to Friday, necessitated by the shortage of nursing staff and a poor bed occupancy rate in the ward.

In December, Miss A. Dunachie reported the following senior nurse appointments:

Deputy	Mrs. G. Pharaoh
for Medical/Elderly services	Mrs. S. Glanz
for Surgical/Rheumatology services	Miss A. Turner

and it was noted all would be in post from mid January, 1987.

Summary of Services

In June, 1986, the West Suffolk Health Authority published a "Summary of Services" in the Authority area and it will be of interest to read a precised extract relating to Newmarket General Hospital.

"Newmarket General Hospital.

Is now a mainly acute hospital with a bed complement of 276. Although there is no Accident and Emergency Department at the hospital, medical, surgical and gynaecological emergencies are admitted directly at the request of General Practitioners; in other specialties the majority of admissions are elective. The Rheumatology Unit at the hospital has been designated as a Regional Demonstration Centre for training, research and development. The hospital is a Training School for State Enrolled Nurses and there are Post Graduate Medical Education facilities on site.

Clinical services include:

Anaesthesia	3 consultants, 1 senior registrar, 1 registrar, 1 part time associate specialist.
E.N.T.	6 beds (2 male Ward C8, 2 female Ward C9, 2 female and children Ward C3), 1 consultant, 1 audiometrician.

Geriatrics	70 beds (Wards B3, B5, B6) and 30 place day hospital. 1 consultant, 1 associate specialist, 3 senior house officers.
Gynaecology	17 beds (Ward C9), 2 consultants, 1 clinical assistant, 3 senior house officers.
Medical	40 beds (19 Ward B1, 21 Ward B2 including 3 coronary care beds), 3 consultants, 1 registrar, 1 senior house officer and 3 house officers (all shared with thoracic medicine and rheumatology).
Neurology	1 Consultant, 1 clinical assistant (outpatient services).
Nursing	general nursing on all wards, outpatient department, geriatric day hospital, x-ray department, theatres, recovery and intensive therapy unit. There is a pupil nurse training school comprising 64 pupils.
Obstetrics	20 beds (Wards A1, A2, A3), 2 consultants, clinical assistants, 2 senior house officers.
Occupational Health	3.5 clinical assistant sessions.
Occupational Therapy	OT for all inpatients, day hospital and consultant outpatient referrals, 5 qualified occupational therapists, 1 aide.
Ophthalmology	2 beds (Ward C3), 1 consultant, orthoptist, ophthalmic optician.
Oral Surgery	4 beds (2 male Ward C6, 2 female Ward C7), 1 consultant, 1 clinical assistant.
Orthopaedics	36 beds (Wards C6 and C7), 4 consultants, 2 senior house officers.
Other Clinical and Clinical Support Services	Chiropody sessions, ECG service, social service department, speech therapy sessions, hospital chaplaincy, surgical appliance fitter, phlebotomy service (for out patients only at present).

Paediatrics	consultant, hospital practitioner.
Pathology	laboratory and post mortem room, 3 consultants, 16.28 medical laboratory scientific officers and technicians, 1 senior post mortem technician, 1.14 outpatient phlebotomist.
Pharmacy	3 pharmacists, 2 technicians, 1 assistant.
Physiotherapy	well equipped department, splint-making and hydrotherapy pool, 13.52 qualified physiotherapists and aides.
Radiology	3 x-ray rooms, 1 ultra sound room, processing facilities, 3 consultants, clinical assistant.
Rheumatology	19 beds (Ward C5), 2 consultants, 1 senior registrar, 1 registrar and 1 senior house officer (both shared with general medicine and thoracic medicine), 1 house officer.
Surgery, General	45 beds (Wards C3, C4, C8), 3 consultants, 1 registrar, 1 senior house officer, 3 house officers.
Theatres	2 main theatres plus 1 theatre for gastroscopies and bronchoscopies, recovery area and 2 bedded intensive therapy unit.
Thoracic Medicine	17 beds (Ward B4), respiratory function laboratory, 1 consultant, 1 registrar, 1 senior house officer (both shared with medical and rheumatology), 1 house officer, 1 clinical assistant.
Voluntary Services	0.5 voluntary services organiser, 40-50 individual volunteers, together with Lions (Hospital Radio), WRVS (coffee shop for outpatients and mobile shop), Red Cross (mobile library, maintenance of flat for relatives) and some 40 volunteer drivers providing transport for visiting relatives."

This gives a pen picture of the situation in mid-1986. It must be remembered that nearly all of the consultant staff were part-time at the hospital, having sessions at other hospitals in Bury St. Edmunds or Cambridge, and the clinical assistant posts would all be sessional and filled by local general practitioners.

1987 Catering Successes and Disappointments

In January, 1987, the League of Friends agreed to buy items of equipment for the hospital, totalling £10,000.

Miss E. J. Woodnough was appointed Sister for Ward B1 from 3rd February and it was noted that Mrs. Orme, the ENB Education Officer, visited and inspected the hospital during the week of 9th February and had subsequently recommended that pupil nurse training should continue for a further two years. It was noted that Mr. C. Constant, the newly-appointed and additional Consultant Orthopaedic Surgeon, would take up his post on 1st May.

Mr. E. Eyre, Catering Manager, resigned on 31st March and Mrs. A. Kallend, Dietitian, had given notice to leave on 10th April. Mr. Eyre was subsequently replaced by Miss Melanie Hogan from 26th May and Mrs. Kallend by Miss Kirsteen Bryson, Senior Dietitian, from 22nd June. Mr. Philip Terry was appointed Staff Pharmacist from 6th July.

Staff Nurse Pryor was appointed Sister for Ward C4 from March. It was noted that the Annual Prizegiving would be held on 3rd April, in the Gibson Centre, when the awards would be presented by Mr. D. Goble, the District Nursing Officer.

During the latter part of 1986 and early into 1987 alterations and upgrading were taking place in the kitchen and it was planned that a trayed meal service for patients would be provided, with central plating and dishwashing. The introduction of this service was delayed until May 1988, when it was introduced with great success.

Hospital staff were affected by a salmonella outbreak in September and four cases were notified. The UMG were concerned that misleading reports in the media apparently caused the Cambridgeshire Social Service department to cancel the regular booking for meals on wheels to be prepared in the hospital kitchen. It was learned later, however, that this was not so: the concern was about the quality of the meals prepared.

In August Catherine Holmes, a feature writer of the Newmarket Journal, asked to undertake a series of features on the work of various departments of the hospital - physiotherapy, occupational therapy, pathology, theatre, catering and works. This move was welcomed and good publicity was gained from the ensuing articles.

B. Johnson, Manager Personnel and Support Services, was selected in November for entry into a management development programme and it was agreed he would transfer to the Health Authority office in Bury St. Edmunds to gain experience there and replace Mr. N. Smith, who would transfer for unit experience to Newmarket General Hospital.

Mrs. B. Newman was appointed Night Nursing Officer from 1st November and Miss Sonia Large, Deputy Medical Records Officer, from 1st December, 1987.

1988 *Continued Support from the Friends and the Newmarket Journal*

The League of Friends again showed great support by agreeing in February to purchase further items of equipment totalling £20,000.

The Annual Prizegiving took place on 4th March in the Gibson Centre when the awards were presented by Mrs. Lesley Williams, Senior Nurse Tutor.

In April it became necessary to close Wards C3 and C8 during the weekends, because of nursing staff shortages. This continued for some months although as staffing became easier it was found possible and economic to close Ward C8 (for general surgery) since there were, generally, not enough patients in the ward during the weekend to justify keeping it open.

In May it was reported that Mrs. G. Pharaoh, Deputy Nursing Manager, had been awarded a travel scholarship of £1,000 by the King's Fund in London to enable her to visit the U.S.A. and study quality issues in hospitals there. The trayed meal service for patients commenced on 23rd May. The unit accountant reported to the UMG an overspend against budget of £109,000.

In August Miss Melanie Hogan, Catering Manager, resigned and it was agreed not to replace her as such but to arrange for Mrs. Lois Grundy, the District Catering Manager, to have overall management responsibility.

Industrial action by the postal services in September caused a repeat of the extraordinary delivery arrangements made in earlier years but all went well with a lot of energy from many members of staff. Sister A. Hipwell was appointed Theatre Sister and Sister Miles, appointed Outpatient Sister, both from 2nd October. It was noted in the same month that Dr. David Stone, Consultant Cardiologist, had been appointed and would be undertaking one session a week at Newmarket General Hospital.

In October Mr. Bull reported to the UMG on the Q.E.D. suggestion scheme and it was agreed to follow this up. In fact, it started on 30th January, 1989 and the first report in February showed that 362 ideas had been put forward by staff to save money and improve the service and some of them looked very promising.

Mrs. Jean Parton was appointed Manager for Midwifery Services for the District on 14th October. The UMG was giving serious consideration to the suggestion of opening a surgical day case ward.

In November the League of Friends ran a Race Night and raised £3,000 towards £4,760 required to purchase a fibrescope required by the anaesthetists: the remainder would come from League funds. An open evening for a 12 week Back to Nursing Course was held on 12th December and the Newmarket Journal Fund raised £2,800 for the purchase of resuscitation training equipment.

1989 *Day Case Ward Opened*

In January, Mr. P. Lester was appointed Catering Manager, accountable to the District Catering Manager. It was reported that at this time the hospital was overspending its budget by nearly £75,000.

In March the Cambridge School of Clinical Medicine gave notice that educational approval for three pre-registration house officer posts would be withdrawn from February, 1990. During this month it became necessary to close the orthopaedic wards because of nursing staff shortages. One bright aspect was that at the end of February the overspending had reduced to £42,000!

In April the hospital incinerator had to be closed down because it no longer complied with the Clean Air Acts and since Crown immunity had been removed it was necessary to make appropriate arrangements with a contractor for the removal of such material, which was very expensive. Responsibility for Newmarket ambulances was switched from Suffolk to Cambridgeshire from 1st April.

In April it was noted that the District hospitals would be taking part in a patient satisfaction survey scheme known as CASPE pat sat, in which five other Districts would be involved. The scheme was programmed to start in November and Miss Julie Cooper was duly appointed the Implementation

Officer. The Medical Staff Committee said farewell to Mr. E. W. Varley, Consultant Oral Surgeon, in April, after 25 years service. He was succeeded by Mr. D. M. Adlam in June.

Meetings in May confirmed that Ward C3 would became a day case ward from October. Staffing levels were agreed as 1 Sister, 4.53 Registered General Nurses (RGN), 4.53 Enrolled Nurses (EN) and 2.25 Auxiliary Nurses (AN), giving 2 RGN, 2EN and 1 AN on duty at all times. It was also noted that in accordance with national developments the Medical Staff Committee at the hospital had expressed an interest to the RHA on their wish to become a NHS Hospital Trust.

Mrs L. Houghton was appointed Hospital Personnel Manager and Mr. W. Higgins, Unit Works Manager, in September. Mr. Eldon Griffiths, MP, paid one of his infrequent visits to the hospital to meet staff on 20th October and Mr. Robinson, Unit Accountant, reported an overspending situation again, with overspending of £48,616 after five months of the year.

Dr. Shneerson started a Sleep Disturbance Clinic session in out-patients in November, in association with ENT consultants. Sessions were held monthly, with six to eight patients. The Royal College of Surgeons' visitor came to the hospital on 18th November and overspending was being reduced: £48,894 after seven months. Mrs. G . Pharaoh, Deputy Nursing Manager, resigned on being promoted to a post with the Kettering Health Authority.

As well as pupil nurse training being carried out at Newmarket, it was pleasing to note that student nurses were returning for part of their RGN training in the wards and departments at the hospital, as well as some of the pupil nurses who were undertaking special training to enable them to take examinations to convert from pupil to state registered nursing.

1990 *Overspending Problems*

In January John Millard was appointed Clinical Nurse Specialist for Operating Theatres/ITU/Recovery. In February it was reported that activity in the day case ward (C3) for the four months to 31st January (apart from the planned four week closure over Christmas and New Year) showed that 299 patients had been cared for.

The Annual Prizegiving for 1990 was held on 6th February at the King Edward Memorial Hall, Newmarket, when Mr. A.S.C. Gibson, JP, was the guest of honour and presented the prizes and awards. This was the last of these occasions as such since from 1991 all hospitals and community staff in the District came together for a whole District Awards Evening, organised by the District Nursing Advisor, Mrs. Kate Wilkinson.

Mr. M.V. Bright was elected Chairman of the Medical Staff Committee and Dr. J. Pearce, Hon. Secretary, and they became the medical representatives on the UMG. Mrs. Moira Newstead and Mrs. Pamela Evans were appointed Clinical Nurse Managers for Medicine & Rheumatology and for the Elderly respectively in March.

Unit overspending at the end of July 1990 was £53,894 for the first four months of the year. In September Mr. Anthony Phillips was appointed Pharmacy Services Manager and Mrs. Patricia O'Sullivan, Assistant General Manager from 15th October.

Nurses and other award winners from Newmarket General Hospital who had not qualified in time for the February occasion, received their awards at the special District evening held at the Corn Exchange in Bury St. Edmunds on 6th September when Mr. Duncan Nicol, CBE, MA, AHSM, Chief Executive of the NHS Management Executive, was the guest of honour.

In November the inspectors of the English National Board visited to examine and review all wards for use in current training of nurses and of two wards with a view to introducing the new training scheme for nurses, Project 2000.

In December the League of Friends agreed a list of purchases put forward by the hospital, amounting to £17,500. Miss Dunachie reported to the UMG a continuing problem with nurse staffing of the medical wards and coronary care unit.

1991 *Maternity Unit Closes*

Notice was received on llth January that the Princess of Wales RAF Hospital in Ely had closed its maternity unit, prior to the Gulf crisis, and that some additional maternity patients would be delivering at Newmarket General Hospital. The overspending at the end of December, 1990, was reported as £57,543 overspent, a reduction of £20,000 over the previous month.

On 22nd February, 1991, the DGM on behalf of the WSHA, issued a consultation document on the future of maternity services at the hospital. It was stated that the provision of these services had been subject to periodic review because of the absence of an associated paediatric unit and the continuously low annual number of deliveries. In 1989 a group of consultants in obstetrics, paediatrics and public health medicine had advised that an associated consultant paediatric unit was essential to provide a safe and acceptable obstetric service and although a service with less than 1500 deliveries a year might be acceptable this would only be so if this was in conjunction with an associated paediatric unit. This unit would need to be on the same site, staffed by preferably three, but at least two consultants, and at least three senior house officers.

The WSHA had decided that the present unit at Newmarket could not comply with these recommendations and, with regret, at its meeting on 28th January had decided to propose closure of the maternity unit to all admissions with effect from 31st July, 1991. The date was selected to give maximum time to make alternative booking arrangements for mothers-to-be due to give birth after that date and to attempt to relieve any anxiety during the waiting period.

Although not the primary cause for the proposed closure, the maternity unit statistics showed that the facilities were not used to the full and the total number of births, even in later years with more admissions from Haverhill and Ely, did not come near the acceptable minimum number of deliveries a year, mentioned above.

Year	Number of Available Beds	Average daily number of beds occupied	Total births
1980	30	11.4	667
1981	30	10.4	637
1982	30	10	651
1983	30	9.7	634
1984	30	8.8	589
1985	30	9.6	587
1986	21	10.9	625
1987	21	10.4	600
1988	21	11.2	685
1989	21	12.1	738

Despite clamour from the local public, indicated on a petition and with many letters of objection, no valid alternative way of meeting these requirements could be found and the unit closed on the due date.

As part of the further reorganisation with the introduction of purchasers and providers and Trusts, discussions were taking place between the District and Unit Managers about future unit shape. It was concluded that from 1st April, 1991, Newmarket General Hospital would merge with the West Suffolk Hospital Unit and some short time after this took place Mr. Eric Bull moved to District HQ in Bury St. Edmunds as Health Contracts Manager for the WSHA, negotiating the purchaser's contract of services with the two units remaining, as well as with other provider units in Cambridge and Norwich.

Mrs. B. Newman, Nurse Manager for Night Duty, retired on 23rd April after 31 years service.

24 Croft Road was sold as surplus to requirements and it was agreed that the income received would be used to purchase additional catering equipment, replacement doors and an extension to the car park.

On 26th April it was reported that the Newmarket Journal Fund had again raised a record sum, of £3,500.

Ward C8 closed on 24th May, following a review of the occupancy of Wards C4 and C8 over the past twelve months from which it was found that there was only 50% occupancy on both wards.

Mrs. Amanda Skull, Manager of the Care of the Elderly at West Suffolk Hospital, assumed managerial responsibility for Newmarket General Hospital. Mr. Gerald Pawsey assumed the financial responsibility as Unit Treasurer, previously carried by Mr. Nigel Robinson. Subsequent changes in the management group meetings were made, allowing for a wider representation to discuss the many and involved operational issues. Meetings were to be held on first and third Fridays monthly with Mr. R.H. Jones (Unit General Manager), Mr. M. V. Bright (Unit Medical Representative), Dr. A. J. Pearce (Hon. Secretary, Medical Staff Committee), Miss A. Dunachie, Mr. G. Pawsey and Mrs. A. Skull present. In addition, a monthly meeting of those listed would be held but with Mrs. A. Fairlay, Personnel Manager and Mr. W. Higgins, Unit Works officer also present.

The District Awards Evening was held on 14th November at the Corn Exchange in Bury St. Edmunds and the Duchess of Norfolk presented prizes and awards.

Miss B. R. Kirk, Manager of the Pathology Laboratory, retired on 15th November and Miss Anne Dunachie accepted early retirement on 31st October in view of the changing nature of the hospital.

1992 Times of Great Change

Although not a popular move, the Assisted Ventilation Unit and Dr. J. Shneerson, vacated its ward and associated accommodation somewhat earlier than planned and expected, and moved, with staff, to Papworth Hospital in February 1992.

On 7th July it was agreed that all acute in-patient admissions would cease from 28th September, 1992 and on 11th September a farewell party was held for staff who were leaving on transfer to other employment in Cambridge or Bury St. Edmunds or taking early retirement or redundancy, since only a limited number of beds for the inpatient elderly, together with out-patient facilities, would remain.

Mr. M. D. Corke, JP, DL, Chairman of the WSHA, who had been associated with health services management in Suffolk for forty-six years was the guest of honour at the District Awards Evening, held in the Corn Exchange in Bury St. Edmunds on 29th September, 1992, when nurses and others from Newmarket and all other hospitals in the District received their awards. A final occasion, with Mr. Corke again presenting the awards, was held in the Cathedral Precinct on 12th March, 1993, three weeks before the Health Authority was amalgamated with East Suffolk Health Authority to form the Suffolk Health Authority.

For the record, officers of the Newmarket Medical Staff Committee during the twelve years 1980 to 1982 were:

	Chairman	Hon. Secretary
1980 - 82	Dr. B. L. Hazleman	Mr. M. V . Bright
1982 - 84	Mr. M. V. Bright	Dr. G.N.W. Kerrigan
1984 - 86	Dr. G.N.W. Kerrigan	Mr. D . J. Dandy
1986 - 88	Mr. D. J. Dandy	Dr. J. Shneerson
1988 - 90	Dr. J. Shneerson	Mr. M. V. Bright
1990 - 92	Mr. M. V. Bright	Dr. A. J. Pearce

Chapter Thirteen

THE CHURCH

The Church was built in 1895 by voluntary contributions raised by members of the Church of England of All Saints, St. Agnes, St. Marys and Exning Churches, with very great success. The following inscription still exists on a stone plaque in the Church:

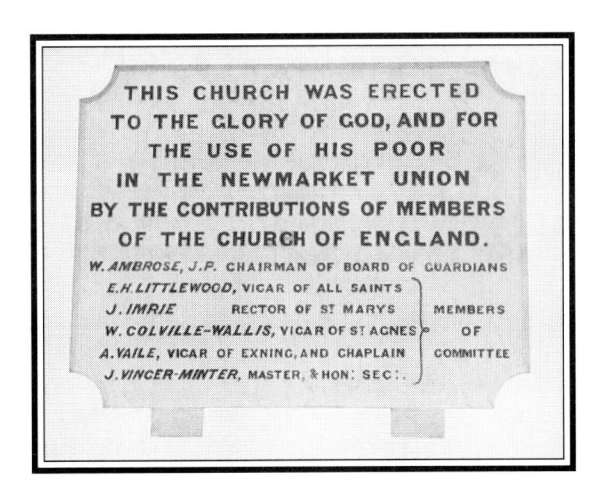

> THIS CHURCH WAS ERECTED
> TO THE GLORY OF GOD, AND FOR
> THE USE OF HIS POOR
> IN THE NEWMARKET UNION
> BY THE CONTRIBUTIONS OF MEMBERS
> OF THE CHURCH OF ENGLAND.
>
> W. AMBROSE, J.P. CHAIRMAN OF BOARD OF GUARDIANS
> E.H. LITTLEWOOD, VICAR OF ALL SAINTS
> J. IMRIE   RECTOR OF ST MARYS
> W. COLVILLE-WALLIS, VICAR OF ST AGNES   MEMBERS OF COMMITTEE
> A. YAILE, VICAR OF EXNING, AND CHAPLAIN
> J. VINCER-MINTER, MASTER, & HON: SEC:

The Church (the Workhouse Chapel), was dedicated to St. Etheldreda on 4th October, 1895 by the Rt. Rev. the Lord Bishop of Ely (Lord Alwyne Compton), assisted by a number of local clergy and at a service attended by a large congregation, which "included in addition to the inmates several of the Board of Guardians and many friends who had taken a kindly and practical interest in the movement for the erection of the Chapel."

The structure of the Church was felt to be a "substantial one" and was considered suitable to seat 250 worshippers. The building contract was carried out by Messrs. Simpson and Son, Exning, on a site donated by the Board of Governors, at a cost of about £500. Various items of furniture were given as gifts by friends.

The list of subscribers to the Chapel Fund shows the considerable local and national interest in the project:

Gift of £100   Mr. H. McCalmont, MP.

Gift of £20	The Jockey Club, Earl of Rosebery, Mr. George Newnes, Bt.
Gift of £10	The Prince of Wales, Duke and Duchess of Portland, Lord Barton, Captain Baird, Messrs. L. de Rothschild, Mr. C.F. Gray and a Miss Chenel for Theatrical Entertainments.
Gift of £5	The Duke of Cambridge, His Excellence the Lord Lieutenant of Ireland, Duke of Westminster, Duchess of Gloucester, Marquis of Bristol, Earl of Ellesmere, Earl of Durham, Lord Bishop of Ely, Countess of Warwick, Countess of Stamford and Warrington, Lord Rothschild, Lord Iveagh, Baron de Hirsch, Lady Wallace, Sir Robert Affleck, Bt., Sir J. Blundell Maple, MP, Hon. W.F.D. Smith, MP, the High Sheriff of Suffolk, Mrs. Gray sen., Mrs. Bulline, Mrs. Scaber, Mrs. Marsh, Messrs. Hanan Bass, MP, Ian Malcolm, MP, Alex Peckover, Daniel Cooper, C.D. Ross, A. M. Ellis, R. Marsh, M.Gurry, Hammond & Co. and Lecture Entertainment (per Hon. Sec.)
Gift of £3	Mrs. L. de Rothschild and Mr. J. A. Dawson.
Gift of £2. 2s. 0d.	Earl of Crewe, Lord Henlipp, Mrs. J. Dawson, Mrs. Bottom, Dr. Maud, Messrs. R.W. King, JP, T. Leader, Foster & Co., J.R. Falder, G. H. Vernall, John Dawson, G. Barrow, A. Slack, F.A. Bainer and H.J. Linzell.
Gift of £2	Rev. E. Case, Mrs. J. Hammond, Miss Stephenson and Mr. G.P. Dawson.
Gift of £1. 1s. 0d.	Dr. Armstead, Mrs. Allix, Mrs. Jennings, Messrs. B. Taylor, B. Stephenson, W. Manning, C.H. Bosworth, Tindall & Co., Bocock and Sons, A. Riley, T. Jennings jun., C. Stebbing and the Gas Company.

In addition to the above monetary gifts, many of the items of furniture and furnishings were donated, viz

Brass Cross	Duchess of Rutland
Altar Frontal	Mrs. D. Cooper
Alms Dish	Rev. Colville Wallis
Paten & Credence table	Mrs. A. M. Ellis
Altar linen	Mrs. Vincer Minter
Altar and Rood screen	Mr. F. Hammond
Challice and Lectern	Rector and Church wardens of St. Mary's
Candlesticks	Rev. A. Barton
Bell	Mr. W. Ambrose, JP, and Mr. Sidney Ennion
Altar hanging	Mrs. E.W. Bard
Altar vases	Rev. E.H. Littlewood
Font	Rev. O. Fisher
Brass Altar desk	Mr. and Mrs. Bridge
Altar lace	Miss Flemington Minter
Altar Service Book	Mr. G.H. Tindall

Local churches offered their church collections at that time which amounted to:

from Gazeley	£1. 12s. 0d.
Exning and St. Philips	£3. 0s. 0d.
St. Mary's, Newmarket	£4. 7s. 6d.
All Saints, Newmarket	£3. 11s. 9d.
Snailwell	10s. 0d.
Borough Green	£1. 0s. 0d.

Whilst the opening portion of the Service of Dedication and the offer of the Dedication Prayer was by the Lord Bishop, attended by his Chaplain, the Rev. E. Bullock Webster, the remainder of the Service was conducted by the Chaplain of the Union, the Rev. A. Vaile, who was the Vicar of Exning and the Chaplain of the Union from 1895 to 1913. The first lesson was read by the Rev. D. Ambrose, Vicar of Teversham, and the second lesson by the Rev. E. H. Littlewood, Vicar of All Saints, Newmarket, and the Rural Dean.

The organist of All Saints, Mr. T. J. Moaksom, "presided at the harmonium" and several members of the Newmarket Philharmonic Band also assisted.

At the conclusion of the Service the Clergy and visitors were entertained to tea in the Boardroom by members of the Building Committee and, in a marquee, loaned by the Jockey Club, the inmates of the Union were treated to "a substantial tea" supplied by Mr. Chennell of the White Hart Hotel.

The day was concluded with a second service in the evening at which the Rev. Canon Cockshott, DD, Vicar of Streatham, Ely, preached to a large congregation. The lessons were read by the Rev. R. C. Allen, Vicar of Whaddon, Bucks, and the Rev. W. S. Eaton, Vicar of St. Philip's.

Other brass plates and plaques in the Church, which still exist, read as follows:

"His Majesty King Edward VII visited this Church July 13th 1904".

"Visit of H.R.H. The Prince of Wales K.G. October 23rd 1895".

"H.R.H. The Duke of Cambridge K.G. attended Service in this Church on Sunday October 23rd 1898".

"DORCAS.
"This woman was full of good works."

Two stained glass windows still exist portraying Queen Victoria and Mrs. Vincer Minter. The inscriptions read:

"This window was erected to the Glory of God and in Memory of Queen Victoria by residents of the neighbourhood - many of the inmates of this Union Home subscribing to the same."

"Queen's shall be thy Nursing Mothers."

"This window is dedicated to the Glory of God and in Memory of Alice Vincer Minter who for 15 years ministered to the comforts of the old folks in this home and interested herself in the beautifying of this Chapel.
Entered into rest Sept. 9th 1904."

There is no doubt the Church played an important part in the daily life of the inmates of the original workhouse and worked closely with Exning Church which was close by but as the role of the Workhouse changed to that of General Hospital its need diminished.

In October 1974 the continued use of the Church was under discussion because the building was underused by patients since, it was said, there were only a limited number of ambulant patients who could make their way there and for the non-ambulant, since it was such a long way from the wards, there were problems with nurses being away from the wards for such a long time. Although a request for use from the parishioners of St. Philips parish was agreed there was little improvement in the attendances and the high cost of maintenance, heating and cleaning made it necessary to consider an alternative use for the building.

The visiting Chaplains agreed that a central counselling room would be much more appropriate and would meet their needs. When this was provided elsewhere it was decided that the Church building could be used as a squash court for hospital staff, which was of particular benefit to resident staff and, in particular, to on-call junior medical staff who could take exercise whilst remaining on site available immediately when required.

It was found that the Church had never been consecrated.

It was eventually agreed, in 1979, with funding from donations and free monies, that a squash court should be built within the walls of the chapel and this was well used, in its early stages.

In 1985 Canon Cedric Catton, Hospital part/time Anglican chaplain, raised with the Health Authority General Manager the possibility of the Authority considering returning the chapel for use as a hospital chapel and, additionally, to replace St. Philips Church, which because of its fabric condition, had a limited life. The Church would refurbish the chapel, if the HA would remove the now underused squash court.

A report on this was given to WSHA on 26 May, 1987 and it was noted that the majority of those using the squash court were friends and relatives of staff, rather than the staff for which it was provided, and that there was an alternative for them just across the road in the leisure centre. The HA agreed in principle to the proposal subject to further discussion and report back.

Although there was some early opposition from staff this was resolved and it was agreed that the chapel would be reinstated from 1st January, 1988, with an annual rent on the lease of site and building, for use by staff, patients and St. Philips' congregation, who would assist in bringing patients from the wards to the church. The Parish agreed to pay the rent, make a donation to the hospital amenity funds and pay for gas services through metering: electricity and water being supplied by the hospital. Two parking places for the chaplains would be provided and preserved. The annual rent would be determined by the District Valuer.

Due much to the effort of Canon Cedric Catton and members of his congregation, The Church of St. Philips w St. Ethelreda was rededicated and licensed by Rt. Rev. John Dennis, Bishop of St. Edmundsbury & Ipswich, at a Sunday evening service on 1st May, 1988. Since a long lease was negotiated it will remain and continue to serve its local hospital and two congregations.

A plaque in the Church commemorates this event:

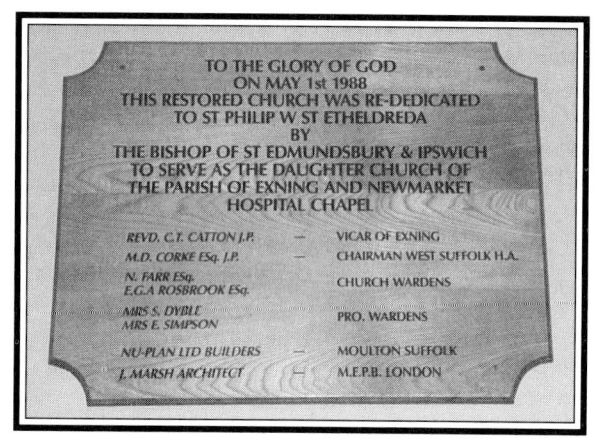

> TO THE GLORY OF GOD
> ON MAY 1st 1988
> THIS RESTORED CHURCH WAS RE-DEDICATED
> TO ST PHILIP W ST ETHELDREDA
> BY
> THE BISHOP OF ST EDMUNDSBURY & IPSWICH
> TO SERVE AS THE DAUGHTER CHURCH OF
> THE PARISH OF EXNING AND NEWMARKET
> HOSPITAL CHAPEL
>
> | REVD. C.T. CATTON J.P. | — | VICAR OF EXNING |
> | M.D. CORKE ESq. J.P. | — | CHAIRMAN WEST SUFFOLK H.A. |
> | N. FARR Esq. E.G.A ROSBROOK Esq. | | CHURCH WARDENS |
> | MRS S. DYBLE MRS E. SIMPSON | | PRO. WARDENS |
> | NU-PLAN LTD BUILDERS | — | MOULTON SUFFOLK |
> | J. MARSH ARCHITECT | — | M.E.P.B. LONDON |

Many of the original artefacts and pews from the Union Church were taken out and spread around other churches in the parish and in Newmarket at the time of change of use but were subsequently recovered and have been restored to the chapel as suitable and appropriate, including the original cross and candles. The pulpit given by the Prince of Wales to the chapel on the occasion of his visit in 1895 is now situated in the Church of St. Nicholas, Landwade, part of the parish of Exning.

Hospital Chaplains who have served since 1895 are:

1895 - 1913	Rev. A. Vaile, Vicar of Exning
1913	Rev. Douglas Hamilton
1927 - 1938	Rev. R. L. Gardener, Vicar of Exning
1938 - 1947	Canon C. Scott, Vicar of Exning
1947 - 1964	Rev. H.A.P. Malachi, Vicar of Exning St. Agnes
1964 - 1982	Canon E. Edmundson, Vicar of Exning
1982 - 1984	Rev. R. Hawkins, Rector of Newmarket
1985 to date	Canon C. T. Catton, Vicar of Exning.

Chapter Fourteen

THE REDEVELOPMENT SAGA

Despite the optimistic references by Dick Heasman in his conclusions, the redevelopment of Newmarket General Hospital became a saga of changing minds and changing circumstances in health care management and not until 1994 was a decision finally obtained and work started! What follows is a severely abbreviated account of activity over a decade to reach this stage.

Members of the West Suffolk Health Authority (WSHA), meeting in January, 1983, received and approved a detailed report from its District Management Team and planners, prepared after many months of discussion with all clinical and other interests at Newmarket General Hospital, entitled "The Redevelopment of Newmarket General Hospital". It pointed out that "a development strategy was now urgently required because some of the existing services were greatly underused and it was increasingly difficult to maintain acceptable standards of care in the antiquated decaying buildings".

An appendix attached to the report on a building condition survey showed that a large proportion, particularly the "B" and "C" Ward blocks, had a limited life expectancy of only a few years.

The Authority agreed that:

(a) the principal role of Newmarket Hospital was as a general hospital supporting West Suffolk Hospital in meeting the health needs of the population of West Suffolk and part of East Cambridgeshire.

(b) provision should be made of a broadly similar range of clinical services to the present with whatever mental illness facilities may be agreed.

(c) there should be a complete redevelopment of buildings and services on the basis of low energy and minimum staffing levels compatible with good practices and the use of technological innovation.

(d) a draft development control plan should be prepared for discussion purposes with a view to agreement and commencement of detailed planning in 1983.

The report and resolutions of the WSHA were passed on to the Regional Health Authority (RHA) and were well received, with a recommendation that the future provision of general surgery and orthopaedic services for the southwest quadrant of the Region should be urgently determined by them. A meeting with the local Community Health Council (CHC) was held on 20th May, 1983, when the report was discussed with its members in some detail.

By February, 1984, service planning aspects of the proposals were being discussed and the RHA confirmed there would be no difficulty in the scheme finding a place in the capital money programme since there was scope for the introduction of new schemes from 1987/88 onwards.

Joint meetings with RHA planning officer teams were held on 19th March, 21st May and 23rd July and in September 1984 a progress report was given to WSHA members. The RHA had decided in December 1983 to locate a "cold" orthopaedic unit at Hinchingbrooke Hospital, Huntingdon, rather than at Newmarket, thus clearing the way for detailed discussions to start on the future reprovision of Newmarket General Hospital. The RHA had confirmed that the case for redevelopment had been accepted in principle and that a joint planning team had been set up to plan a hospital of 355 beds (205 acute, 30 obstetric, 96 geriatric and 24 psychogeriatric).

This continued to be the basis of planning and provision was made in the RHA capital programme to earmark monies to start rebuilding in 1987/88. Detailed planning work followed.

In January, 1987, the RHA decided to enquire by way of a southwest quadrant option appraisal, what health care facilities needed to be available to meet the needs of the population served by Newmarket, Cambridge and Huntingdon (the southwest quadrant of the region). This dramatically delayed the further planning and start of building for Newmarket since it was argued that not until the option appraisal outcome was apparent should any start be made.

By October 1988, following the completion of the option appraisal and consideration of its findings, the RHA had accepted that acute services should be redeveloped at Newmarket General Hospital. As part of an exercise to determine the amount of accommodation to be provided in an enlarged Addenbrooke's Hospital, regional officers investigated an increased service at Newmarket and Ely.

Medical staffing problems at Newmarket were not helping the situation. In December the University of Cambridge School of Clinical Medicine gave only limited twelve months approval for house surgeon posts and it was later reported that from February, 1990, this approval (for three house officer posts) would be withdrawn. On 18th April, 1989, the District General Manager had a meeting with all consultant surgical staff concerning the future of general surgery at Newmarket and, by implication, at the West Suffolk Hospital, particularly in view of CEPOD (Confidential Enquiry into Peri-operative Deaths). This stipulated that it was not acceptable to have emergency admissions of general surgical and urological cases at both sites without consultant staff being available at both. Hitherto the consultant was on duty covering both sites, which had produced some problems when he was occupied with emergency operating theatre work at one hospital, but required also at the other.

By the end of 1988 agreement had been reached between Cambridge and West Suffolk Health Authorities that an additional 48 beds above the catchment population demands would be added to Newmarket bed complement. By this time the planning and site appraisal had been completed for the new development but, at this late stage, the viability of acute inpatient services at Newmarket came into question again because of CEPOD and a Department of Health medical staffing requirement publication "Achieving a Balance", which called for reassessment.

On 6th September, 1989, the RHA created a Regional Working Group with a remit to recommend to the RHA in October a new replacement hospital at Newmarket containing major outpatient facilities, major day treatment/day surgery facilities, an inpatient unit of 90 - 100 beds for the elderly, some provision of general practitioner beds and with purpose planned and built facilities to be provided on site, with private nursing home/facilities on the same site (to be administered privately).

Members of the Working Group included Mr. M. V. Bright, Dr. J. Shneerson, Dr. J. Calvert and Dr. S. Bailey (general practitioners) from Newmarket, Dr. R. West, Consultant in Public Health Medicine and Mr. J. R. Melleney, District General Manager, from WSHA, Dr. R. Zimmern, Consultant in Public Health Medicine, Cambridge HA, Dr. J.P. Hutchby, Consultant in Public Health Medicine, EARHA and Mr. W.A.B. Smellie, Consultant Surgeon representing the Royal College of Surgeons.

At its first meeting the remit was challenged by the DGM, with considerable support from the clinicians present, and an additional item was added "to review these in the light of the other major options and make recommendations."

Six meetings were held between 16th September and 17th October, 1989 and these were long, tortuous and on some occasions, quite acrimonious. Members met with a number of specialists relating to day surgery, obstetrics, general and orthopaedic surgery and radiology.

The Working Group concluded that there were three options to be considered, viz:

(a) as a community hospital acute services being redistributed in West Suffolk and Cambridge Health Districts.

(b) redevelopment as an acute hospital of 400 beds (SW option appraisal preferred option).

(c) redevelopment as an acute hospital of 600 beds.

It was agreed that the 600 bed acute hospital option (c) could not be justified in terms of the projected population to be served. Although the population could possibly sustain an option (b) hospital of 400 beds (275 acute) this would provide insufficient workload to justify the additional numbers of medical staff required to comply with CEPOD and "Achieving a Balance". It was reluctantly concluded, therefore, that only the community hospital option (a) was a viable option, providing highly effective outpatient and diagnostic services for acute specialties (with open access to general practitioners), inpatient and day facilities for geriatric and ESMI (psychogeriatric) patients.

The final report was prepared for the RHA meeting on 22nd November and its author, because it was not a unanimous view, concluded that the redevelopment of the hospital as a "community" hospital was now the only viable option. This followed particularly further appraisal against agreed national principles for improving patient safety in the peri-operative period (CEPOD Report) and Department of Health medical staffing requirements under "Achieving a Balance".

Sir Eldon Griffiths, MP, on reading of these conclusions, declared his intent to fight for Newmarket General Hospital to retain its acute hospital status. He held public meetings in Exning and meetings with hospital staff in the Gibson Centre during November. Mr. James Paice, MP, and Mrs. Gillian Shepherd, MP, from adjacent constituencies pledged their support to ensure appropriate hospital services for their constituents.

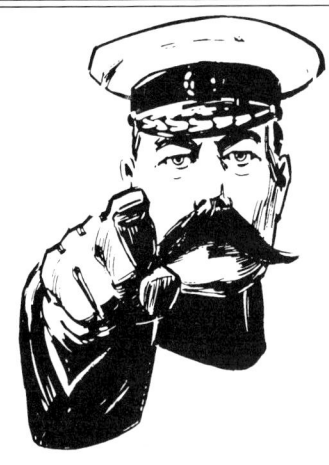

YOUR HOSPITAL NEEDS YOU NOW.

ONCE AGAIN IT URGENTLY REQUIRES A "LIFE SUPPORT SYSTEM"

JOIN THE FIGHT FOR ITS LIFE TODAY, IT COULD SAVE YOURS TOMORROW

CAMPAIGN FOR NEWMARKET GENERAL TO BE REBUILT AS A FULLY OPERATIONAL HOSPITAL COMPLETE WITH ITS MATERNITY UNIT

Printed and issued by Anglia Windscreens Ltd

Campaign Poster

Despite enormous opposition to these conclusions the RHA decided during January and February, 1990, to produce a consultation paper on all aspects of the southwest quadrant appraisal to cover future development of facilities at Newmarket, Addenbrooke's, Papworth and Hinchingbrooke Hospitals. This was eagerly awaited but was never published, as such, since at the April 1990 meeting the RHA decided that each of the District Health Authorities involved (West Suffolk, Cambridge and Huntingdon) should produce its own consultative document. This was most frustrating since this was the obvious line which had been suggested to the RHA, three months earlier!

Sir Eldon, supporting as President a local campaign group for the retention of Newmarket General Hospital, raised questions in the House of the Secretary of State about the national norm of the minimum number of acute beds and the status of CEPOD and "Achieving a Balance" and in his terrier-like fashion had a lengthy correspondence with the Secretary of State and the civil service.

On 10th May, 1990, the Medical Staff Committee gave an assurance that there was total professional commitment by the consultant staff to maintain and develop the acute services at Newmarket into the new hospital. They warned that prolonged further delay would lead to rapidly increasing difficulties in providing safe patient care. It was noted that Royal College of Surgeons approval for junior medical staff training was now limited to six months: this decision would be reviewed further and approval would be continued if there was demonstrable improvement in supervision and training aspects covering the posts.

The RHA required WSHA to consult widely on the future role of Newmarket General Hospital as the basis for redevelopment and whilst agreeing that the form of the consultation paper should be decided by the WSHA there were to be four major constraints, viz

    (a) any option to retain acute inpatient services must be substantiated by clear purchasing intention of the relevant District Health Authorities and General Practitioners.

    (b) any intention to retain acute inpatient services would need to take account of medical staffing contracts imposed by CEPOD and "Achieving a Balance" and the recognition of training posts in medical posts.

    (c) conclusions must take account of RHA statement of values and principles and the requirements of undergraduate teaching and medical research.

    (d) the consultation should be with all interested parties.

To assist their case, the Committee for the Retention of Newmarket General Hospital commissioned private consultants, Paul Cooper & Associates, who produced a report "The case for immediate redevelopment as an acute hospital" claiming to identify and produce an independent review of the principal options for the provision of hospital services in the southwest quadrant of the East Anglia region.

The WSHA consultation document "The Future of Newmarket General Hospital" was published on 24th July, 1990, to a meeting of Authority members, with special invitations to Medical Staff Committee Chairmen (of the District Medical Committee, Newmarket and West Suffolk Hospital Medical Staff Committees), to the Chairman of the Committee for the Retention of Newmarket Hospital (Mr. K. Kemp-Turner) and the Chairman and Secretary of the West Suffolk Community Health Council (Mr. H. Place and Mrs. R. Shadbolt).

Following this meeting the DGM on 26th July, 1990, wrote to the Regional General Manager with a full and detailed case from WSHA, with their views and recommendations which, summarised, amounted to:

1. the WSHA reaffirmed its previous and long-held view (since 1983) that Newmarket General Hospital should be redeveloped to 400 beds (250 acute) with full outpatient and diagnostic services, etc.

2. because of population projections and uncertainties of the White Paper market conditions to apply from April 1991, a special case should be made for additional funding to meet the costs of these and for CEPOD and "Achieving a Balance" and for medical staffing approvals without detriment to present or future levels of services provided by West Suffolk Hospital.

On 17th September, 1990, the Authority membership changed as a result of the Government's White Paper "Working for Patients" and the NHS and Community Care Act. The former eighteen members were replaced by a new Authority, composed of a Chairman (Mr. M. D. Corke), five non-executive members and five executive members (the former Management Board members). The Chairman and four of the non-executive members (Mr. D. Barnard, Mrs. S. Tamlyn, Mrs. R. Varley and Mr. S. Whitwell) were reappointed to membership, along with a new member Mr. E. Flack. Chief Officers remained, but with some new titles, as Chief Executive Mr. J.R. Melleney, Director of Finance & Information Mr. G. C. Elliot, Director of Planning &

Personnel Mrs. J. Rutherford, Director of Public Health Dr. R. West and Chief Nursing Advisor Mrs. K. Wilkinson.

It came as no surprise when on 27th September the RHA responded advising the WSHA that it could not agree to make or support extra funding or medical staff post approvals which would be contrary to the objectives and the spirit of the NHS reform, due from 1st April, 1991. Providing extra funding, bypassing the purchaser concept, would totally undermine the key aim of the reforms of achieving better value for money.

A press release, causing concern and some anger amongst those involved in this protracted situation who read it, advised the media that the requests had been turned down and that "the WSHA had been told to think again about its plans for Newmarket Hospital. Proposals to redevelop must be based on clear evidence that they would be financially viable and if this cannot be done it should pursue other options such as its redevelopment as a community hospital."

Sir Eldon Griffiths, MP, was one of those angered by the apparent rebuke to his local Health Authority.

At its meeting on 22nd October, 1990, members of the WSHA received full reports on the situation to date and, in particular, that the Newmarket Medical Staff had once again rejected an option to maintain the status quo at Newmarket for a further five years, to give time for the reform effects to be more accurately measured, so that the only option now available was to consult on the provision of the community hospital solution.

Members were concerned that they were being asked to identify clear purchasing intentions for the services of Newmarket Hospital in a climate when market conditions could not be predicted and expressed their dissatisfaction with the situation whereby the RHA were forcing them to pursue an option with which they did not agree. After lengthy discussion, during which the paramount importance of the need to dispel the uncertainty of staff at the hospital about their future was reaffirmed, members voted on and by a majority approved the following resolution:

> "Following the RHA's refusal to adopt and fund the recommendations agreed at the meeting of the former West Suffolk Health Authority on 24th July, 1990, the Health Authority reluctantly has no alternative but to go out to consultation on the proposal to redevelop Newmarket Hospital as a community hospital."

In November, 1990, this further consultation document "The Development of Newmarket General Hospital as a Community Hospital" was published and was issued for public consultation on 3rd December.

In this document the WSHA explained not only what its intentions were so far as the community hospital were concerned, but spelled out in some detail the changed circumstances and the uncertainties caused by the changes which had, to an extent, forced its hand.

In a section on its strategic objectives it pointed out that Health Authorities' strategic objectives had been affected by the Government's White Paper "Working for Patients" which imposed on them a principal responsibility for purchasing health care for their resident population, while continuing to manage (before NHS Trusts were formed) facilities and services within the District. New funding arrangements on a weighted capitation basis would come into formal operation from 1st April, 1991.

It pointed out that the implications for Newmarket General Hospital, with its catchment area spanning two health authority boundaries, would be that its existence would depend on contracts to provide care from the two respective authorities and, to a lesser extent (14% of the total workload in 1988/89), from other Districts within and outside of East Anglia. It argued that under-utilised facilities would not be funded directly by any one authority but that the overhead costs of these facilities would be borne on a proportionate basis by all of the purchasers: at a higher rate than would be the norm. There would be doubt as to whether purchasers would be prepared to continue to fund this spare capacity in this way. Making the situation even more complex, this spare capacity could not be taken up without significant extra numbers of senior medical staff, which could not be justified.

In February, 1991, the Committee for the Retention of Newmarket Hospital, who had employed a second private company of management consultants, J. J. Thompson & Partners, published their advisors' report "The Case for retaining acute services at Newmarket General Hospital". This report was presented and discussed informally by Mr. Kemp-Turner and Thompson representatives with the Chairman and Chief Officers of the WSHA on l5th March and a special private meeting of the WSHA was held a week later to give preliminary consideration to the comments received on the consultation document and on the Thompson report.

At the public meeting of the WSHA, held on 25th March, 1991, the comments received on the consultation document, the Thompson report and the views of the West Suffolk Community Health Council were discussed. After a long debate the members unanimously adopted the resolution:

> "It was proposed that since neither the Health Authority nor, in the opinion of the Health Authority, the Community Health Council and the Committee for the Retention of Newmarket General Hospital, had been able to find a way to overcome the medical staffing problems, future revenue funding and the guaranteed viability of Newmarket General Hospital in its new provider role from 1st April, the Health Authority had no alternative but to recommend to the Regional Health Authority that the hospital should be replaced by a new community hospital. This should contain the best possible level of health care accommodation and facilities commensurate with its size and location and it, together with the additional in-patient accommodation and support services at the West Suffolk and Addenbrooke's Hospitals, should be provided at the earliest possible opportunity in the capital programme."

The DGM, in his letter of 2nd April to the RHA conveying this decision, advised that the Community Health Council did not support this decision and would be making an appeal against it in due course. He also asked that the RHA should consider this matter as a matter of urgency since they would be well aware of all the anxieties and uncertainties that had prevailed for many years on the future of the hospital and its effect on staff morale and public confidence. Further delay would merely exacerbate the situation and make the task of retaining acute services at Newmarket, during the period of rebuilding, that much more difficult.

Clearly, too, this decision was not acceptable to the people of Newmarket. A massive petition was prepared and handed in to the Prime Minister's office on 15th May and more than 9,000 people marched through the town centre on 19th March in protest at the Health Authority plans.

The RHA did not consider this matter until its June meeting, needing the extra time to carry out more detailed work on the presentation of information, particularly in the light of purchasing authority intentions under the options and of the views obtained from the consultation. In the event, the RHA endorsed the recommendation and passed it through to the Secretary of State for Health in July, 1991.

Showing some anxiety about the outcome of all this Mr. Kemp-Turner, on behalf of his Committee, wrote to the Secretary of State for Health on 19th June, expressing an interest in sponsoring an application for NHS Trust status for Newmarket Hospital. Sir Eldon Griffiths wrote a week later to the Secretary of State supporting this application which he "had read with interest and complete agreement."

So far as the public were concerned all then went quiet but, of course, there was much activity at the RHA and at the Department of Health.

On 22nd January, 1992, with still no decision from the Secretary of State, the DGM attended a meeting of the Newmarket Medical Staff Committee to discuss with clinicians the practicalities of maintaining acute services whilst awaiting the decision and, if it became necessary, how to make a planned and orderly withdrawal of services and for their reprovision at the West Suffolk and Addenbrooke's Hospital.

The Secretary of State's decision was announced on 10th February, 1992, in letters to the Chairmen of the RHA and WSHA from Mr. Stephen Dorrell, Parliamentary Under Secretary of State for Health. In this letter he gave general support to the conclusions concerning the community hospital provision but questioned the range of services and asked the WSHA to consider the provision of a general practitioner/midwife maternity unit, a minor casualty unit and day surgery facilities, although it was agreed that planning could proceed on this basis with the condition that the three issues were examined and reports submitted to Ministers.

The RHA, WSHA and Cambridge HA all expressed views on this decision as did the local Member of Parliament and all were delighted that a decision had been reached - although not all thought the decision was correct - at last putting an end to the long period of uncertainty and anxiety for patients and staff. It was confirmed that the RHA had earmarked £18m. for the new hospital and £6m. for the additional beds and facilities at the West Suffolk and Addenbrooke's Hospitals providing inpatient care for Newmarket residents.

Over the next three months intensive consultation took place with all interests, particularly with hospital medical staff and general practitioners, on the three proposals. A detailed report was produced for the WSHA meeting in June 1992 and the RHA was subsequently informed that a decision on the maternity unit had not been reached since a public meeting was to be held, but that the Authority could not support a minor casualty unit, but would maintain diagnostic and treatment departments for general practitioner access, and provision for day surgery and outpatient procedures would be included in the new hospital, as had always been the intention.

In a follow up letter, the RHA were advised on 27th July that after holding a public meeting to learn from the community what maternity services it wanted, the WSHA did not consider it practicable from a safety or financial viability point of view to include a general practitioner/midwife obstetric unit within the community hospital. It was confirmed that the ante- and post-natal services would be maintained and enhanced and, meeting the public request, the Authority would attempt to enhance the "domino" maternity service for patients with more home delivery and, where considered appropriate, delivery in the acute hospital with the domiciliary midwife present.

These conclusions were endorsed by the RHA and, in due course, accepted by Ministers.

On 22nd June, a Steering Group of officers for the Newmarket Community Hospital redevelopment was set up: the outline functional content was prepared, the intentions of the purchasing authorities obtained and design work commenced. This stage then allowed the Steering Group to be disbanded and the project team formed.

Plans were announced in June, 1992, for the run-down of acute services at Newmarket and the smooth transfer of services and the maintenance of high quality care of those remaining inpatients and of those who would be admitted to West Suffolk and Addenbrooke's Hospital in future for acute care. It was agreed that transfers would take place, when additional or new facilities were created, as follows:

General medicine	West Suffolk/Addenbrooke's	8 June 1992
Chest medicine	West Suffolk	8 June 1992
Coronary care	West Suffolk	8 June 1992
Urology	West Suffolk	8 June and 28 September 1992
Oral Surgery	Addenbrooke's	14 September 1992
Orthopaedic surgery	Addenbrooke's	14 September 1992
Gynaecology	West Suffolk/Addenbrooke's	21 September 1992
General surgery	West Suffolk/Addenbrooke's	28 September 1992
Acute geriatric	West Suffolk/Addenbrooke's	28 September 1992
Rheumatology	Addenbrooke's	28 September 1992
ENT	Addenbrooke's	28 September 1992
Day Surgery	West Suffolk (new unit)	Spring 1993
	Addenbrooke's	September 1992

and transfers took place, more or less, on these dates.

In March 1993 the WSHA formally approved the proposal that the management of Newmarket General Hospital and its redevelopment should become the responsibility of the Mid Anglia Community Health NHS Trust (formerly the Community Unit) from 1st April, 1993, on an agency basis for the Suffolk Health Authority. Newmarket formally transferred to the Trust on 1st April, 1994, having been managed by the West Suffolk Hospitals Unit from May 1991 to March 1993.

On 31st March, 1993, the West Suffolk Health Authority was dissolved on amalgamation with East Suffolk to form the Suffolk Health Authority.

The Mid Anglia Community Health NHS Trust was formed from 1st April 1993 and Mrs. Rosie Varley, a former member and Vice Chairman of the WSHA, was appointed its Chairman.

At a formal presentation held in the Gibson Centre on 23rd February, 1994, Mrs. Varley announced that the Secretary of State had given approval for the construction of a purpose-built community hospital for Newmarket, at a total capital cost of £8m., allowing the Trust to press ahead with the implementation of its well publicised commitment to develop community services for local people. A business case for the new development had been approved in November, 1993, and the new hospital would be built in three phases, the first construction work starting in December 1994. This stage would contain 23 beds for the elderly patient (for rehabilitation and respite care), 6 beds for general practitioner patients, a day centre of 15 places for the elderly, a day centre of 12 places for the elderly mentally infirm, together with new physiotherapy and occupational therapy departments.

Later phases, which it was hoped would be built consecutively, but in the event have been merged so that there will be only two phases, would provide a new outpatient department, administration, a resource centre, medical records department, a minor treatment room, pathology, pharmacy, refurbishment of the X-ray Department, a mental health resource centre and accommodation for works, stores and catering. It is expected that all phases would be completed by September, 1996 and commissioned for use shortly thereafter.

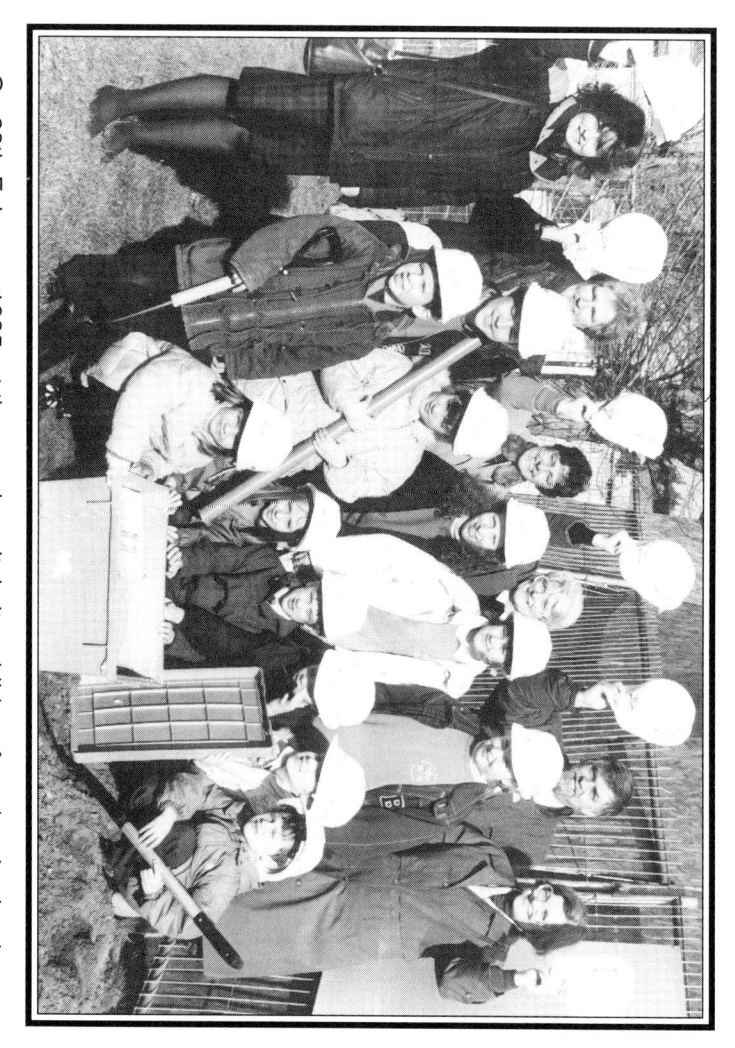

On 28th February 1995, at the new hospital site, children from local schools and hospital staff buried time capsules containing items that will give future generations an insight of life in Newmarket in the 1990s. The capsules will remain unopened for at least 50 years.

Photograph reproduced with the kind permission of Paul Hammond (Newmarket Journal)

Chapter Fifteen

TABULATED HISTORY OF NEWMARKET GENERAL HOSPITAL

1830 The Guardians of the Newmarket Union of Parish Houses decided there was a need for a central Union or Workhouse in Newmarket.

1835 Meetings commenced in Kingston House rooms, Newmarket.

1836 The Newmarket Guardians recommended the purchase of four acres of land at a cost not exceeding £400 and for a Workhouse to be built, the cost not to exceed £7,500. Work started in June, 1836. Mr. A. Charles Guy was appointed Master.

1840 Board of Guardians introduced vaccination against smallpox for all persons residing in the Workhouse.

1850 Gas jet lighting being introduced.

1875 Terraced houses adjoining the Workhouse in Gwynne Terrace built.

1889 Mr and Mrs Vincer Minter appointed Master and Matron.

1890 The Hospital Church built from voluntary contributions raised by members of other Church of England Churches in the town.

Infirmary wards built in line with the Act of 1867.

1911 Mr. E. S. Heasman appointed Master.

1912 Mrs. A. V. Heasman appointed Matron.

1929 Responsibilities transferred to Local Authorities. Newmarket Workhouse came under the control of West Suffolk County Council. The name was changed to Newmarket Public Assistance Institution. The Board of Guardians was dissolved and House Committees appointed.

1932 Care and teaching of children ceased. General improvements started, ceilings fitted to open roofs, wood block floors laid, a form of steam heating started to be installed. Washing machines and hydro extractor fitted in laundry. Programme of replacing iron windows with wood and curtains fitted.

1935   Installation of electric lighting and power.

1936   New nursery built. Accommodation in "A" Block let to Newmarket Rural District Council as offices.

1938   The Ministry of Health made a general survey of the Institution and grounds.

1939   The Newmarket Public Assistance Institution designated as an Emergency Medical Services Hospital. The name was changed to White Lodge Emergency Hospital. Inmates transferred to other Institutions in the county. Colonel Watson and Miss Lithgow arrived to be Medical Superintendent and Matron of the new hospital. Experienced medical and nursing staff arrived. Casual or tramp wards closed.

1940   All the original accommodation for E.M.S. use. Air raids started in April. Military casualties, from the Dunkirk evacuation, arrived between May and June. Dining hall in "A" Block divided to form a temporary outpatient department. Decision made that a further nine wards were required ("C" Block) to include X-ray department, theatres, kitchens, mortuary and boiler house plant. One and a half acres of adjoining paddocks requisitioned. Present sisters changing room in "A" Block used as temporary x-ray room. Agreed the day to day management of the hospital should continue under a sub-committee of the West Suffolk County Council Public Assistance Department as agent for the Ministry of Health in Cambridge. Entrance hut and iron gates and railings removed to make bombs. Pony tub cart and pony sent to Sudbury Public Assistance Institution.

1941   Newmarket High Street bombed and casualties admitted. Tramp ward accommodation converted into A.R.P. and decontamination centre. Six new wards in "B" Block opened in February 1941. Edward Ward, at present part of the maternity department, used as a resuscitation room. Children transferred to other Institutions and the nursery converted to massage and physiotherapy department. Large American steam operated drum sterilizer installed in "C" Block. Fire watchers recruited from hospital staff. Major Albury appointed Military Registrar for the Cambridge group. Messrs. Kings of Exning started building new pack store and mortuary in "C" Block. Dr. Morrey appointed pathologist. Electric power installed in laundry. Three members of the medical staff recruited from the West London Teaching Hospital, Hammersmith.

1942 Enquiry office and telephone kiosk built in entrance hall of "A" Block. Cleveland House, Newmarket, requisitioned and used to accommodate 25 nurses. Mrs. A. V. Heasman retired 17th January, 1942, owing to ill health. Mr. E. S. Heasman appointed Clerk and Steward. "C" Block opened in February, beds increased to 700. Ministry of Health requested ward to be set aside for children, ground floor of Ward A3 used for this purpose. Miss M. Welply appointed House Surgeon in February. Mr. G. Thompson appointed Pharmacist. Occupational therapy and remedial medicine department opened. Air raids on Norwich in April. 175 patients admitted from Norfolk and Norwich Hospital. "C" kitchen opened in March. New boiler house and mortuary opened in April. A trailer fire pump obtained and staff trained in its use. Red Cross library opened. Staff entertainment committee formed and regular concerts given for patients. Public performance given in the Turner Hall, Newmarket, in November 1943. ENSA concerts started. Pathology department recognised as Area Laboratory. Pack store, for clothing of service patients, opened in August. Military Registrars office opened. St. Phillips Hall used as a recreational hall for service patients. Small military police force attached to the hospital. Heathfield House, Newmarket, requisitioned in September for patients' rehabilitation. New nurses' home opened in "C" Block. Application to open Nurses' Training School refused by the General Nursing Council. Dr. Platts joined the hospital staff from the West London Teaching Hospital.

1943 Dental centre opened. Mr. E. S. Jamieson took over fracture department on 28th August. Physiotherapy department started short courses for masseurs in rehabilitation. Remainder of adjoining paddock requisitioned by the Ministry of Health. It was not handed over to the hospital until June 1944. Laundry upgraded - Cochran boiler house built. Wards B4 and B6 set aside for TB patients. 6 small chalets purchased and open verandahs built on wards B2, B4, B6. In October the Ministry of Health made the hospital a receiving centre for TB patients from other hospitals in the area.

1944 Oakfield House, Newmarket, de-requisitioned by Air Ministry. Application for use by the hospital was refused. 26 children from a children's hospital in Walsham le Willows admitted following an outbreak of gastro-enteritis - two died in hospital. Major Bailey Hawkins took over the duties of transport officer.

1945 Osborne House, Newmarket, used a nurses' home. Mr. Bertie Newton died in the Board Room following a heart attack. A shelter for the patients in "C" Block built on land at the back of the laundry. The first Hospital Open Day was held on 1st July. The Army withdrew the ambulance service in June. Some old converted ambulances and cars obtained from the Civil Defence. Parker's Garage in Field Terrace Road purchased. The American ambulance service based at Cambridge closed down. Permission to remove the air raid shelters was refused by the War Office. Leys School, Cambridge, closed down - orthopaedic and nerve injury cases transferred to Newmarket General Hospital. The buildings used as A.R.P. and contamination centre handed back to the hospital by Civil Defence. The name of the hospital changed to White Lodge Hospital. On 25th September the Ministry of Health ruled that White Lodge Hospital should work independently of Addenbrooke's Hospital. The Deans x-ray unit was replaced by a new Westinghouse unit, ex lease lend. The general practitioners were notified that the hospital was open for regular admission of certain classes of civilian patients.

1946 A large number of nursing staff applied for release. Oakfield House was handed back to the owners on 19th June. Heathfield House and Cleveland House, de-requisitioned and handed back to the owners in May. Nursery for children, under two years, opened for the West Suffolk County Council. Miss Lithgow resigned her post of Matron in September. Miss Finch appointed Matron in September, resigning in December 1946. Miss S. M. Hay appointed Matron. The General Nursing Council authorised White Lodge Hospital to be a Training School for Assistant Nurses. St. Fabians estate purchased in November. Ward A1 converted into a maternity unit in December.

1947 All military staff withdrawn from the hospital, duties transferred to the Clerk and Steward. Colonel Watson retired 18th March. Air Vice Marshal T. Kelly, CBE, MC, MD, appointed Medical Superintendent 29th August. Unit for the late treatment of poliomyelitis opened, Mr. E. S. Jamieson in charge. Ward C1 converted to outpatient department.

1948 The National Health Service introduced in July. East Anglian Regional Hospital Board (No.4) formed to administer the hospital services in East Anglia. South West (No. 1) Group Hospital Management Committee based at White Lodge Hospital: Chairman, Captain H. R. King, CBE, JP. The hospital administrative duties of the West Suffolk County Council ceased. The training school for nurses commenced.

1950 Mental and psychiatric hospitals withdrawn and formed separate No. 13 Hospital Management Committee Group, based at Fulbourn Hospital.

1951 Mr. E. S. Heasman, Clerk and Steward retired, duties being taken over by the Group Secretary Brigadier T. R. Henry. Dr. Charles Hay took over the chest clinic from Dr. Arden Jones. The name of the hospital was changed to Newmarket General Hospital.

1952 The Hospital's first Nurses' Prizegiving held.

1954 The General Nurse Training School established at St. Fabians estate. Miss Spiller appointed Sister Tutor. Nurses recruitment drives held in the Newmarket, Haverhill, Soham and Cambridge areas. Advertisement on Anglia television. Cardigan Street nurses' home, Newmarket, used as a maternity unit, staffed from main hospital. Staff recreational bus service to Cambridge started. Hospital fire services improved in conjunction with County and Newmarket Fire Brigades. New 100 line telephone exchange installed. The Group Secretary, Brigadier Henry retired, being succeeded by Mr. A. W. Youngs. The Nurses' Training School badge was adopted as the Hospital Badge. Cross infection committee set up in May. TV sets started to be introduced into the wards. The Bishop of St. Edmundsbury & Ipswich presented prizes at the Nurses' Prizegiving and opened an extension to the patients' pillow radio service from the Church. Renovations to the Maternity unit started in September. The Hospital cricket team won the Pudney Cup Cricket competition. The laundry services for all the hospitals in the Group centralised at Newmarket General Hospital. Improvements to laundry including building a new central linen store and sewing room.

1955 Major upgrading work started on the main kitchen in "C" Block. Staff central dining room opened in "C" Block. Group Medical Advisory Committee formed. Mr. J. Rowlands resigned in April being succeeded by Mr. R. E. B. Tagart, Consultant Surgeon. Patients' call system extended to all wards. Air Vice Marshal Kelly retired in November and Medical Superintendent duties taken over by Mr. R. Williamson, Consultant E.N.T. Surgeon on a part-time basis. Dr. I.P. Williams was appointed Consultant Radiologist. The services of the pathology, theatre and x-ray departments extended to provide 24 hour cover. A 16mm training film made by the Physiotherapy Department with the help of the Photography Department at Addenbrooke's Hospital.

1956   2¼ acres of land at St. Fabians estate sold to the West Suffolk County Council for the present Upper School to be built. The first annual Hospital Ball was held in the Memorial Hall, Newmarket. A two-way arrangement for the admission of medical patients was agreed with Addenbrooke's Hospital. "C" Block corridor enclosed in May. Daily living unit opened as part of the Occupational Therapy Department.

1957   A campaign to recruit nursing auxiliaries from Spain started. The senior house officer posts in Orthopaedics and General Surgery recognised by the Royal College of Surgeons of England as qualifying training posts for the Fellowship examinations of the College. GPO mobile telephone service introduced in the TB wards.

1958   Staff hard tennis court provided at St. Fabians. 44 hour week introduced for nursing and midwifery staff.

1959   Service lift between ground and first floor of maternity unit installed. Scheme for annual x-rays of all nursing staff introduced. Dr. J. H. Dean, Consultant Pathologist, appointed Control of Infection Officer. Multitone pocket paging system for nominated staff introduced. Standby electric generator installed for boiler house, theatre and portable x-ray machine. Mr. Thorborne appointed Hospital and Group Catering Officer.

1960   RHB training scheme for medical laboratory technicians started. A new 100 line telephone exchange installed with direct dialling of all internal calls. Hydrotherapy pool opened in July.

1961   Six new staff garages opened at St. Fabians. The first ward clerks appointed. Mr. R. Williamson, Consultant ENT Surgeon and part-time Medical Superintendent retired. Duties of Medical Superintendent taken over by Dr. A. Robertson, Consultant Anaesthetist. The General

Nursing Council withdrew approved for general nurse training school. A preliminary training school was opened in "A" Block. The colours of the Hospital Badge were changed. St. Fabian House used as a Sisters' Home. "B" Block corridor enclosed.

1962   The first annual Hospital Ball was held at Soham. Local family planning clinics started in Newmarket in January. Work study on hospital portering service completed. White Cottage at St. Fabians demolished in September. Patients' choice of menu introduced in April. Training scheme for apprentice cooks introduced and renewal of electrical and mechanical services started. Wards modified to provide dayrooms. Stephen Lycett Green, Chairman of the East Anglian Regional Hospital Board, opened Oakfield House as a nurses' home. A start was made on providing disposeable bed pan units in the wards. Two new medical staff flats opened at St.Fabians in November and two cottages and gardens at St. Fabians were sold to the West Suffolk County Council.

1963   A NO SMOKING rule in corridors and wards introduced. Work study on hospital domestic services started and ward and department top-up linen service introduced in June. New boiler house in "C" Block opened in January and replacement electrical and mechanical services completed by November. Enrolled Nurse Training School replaced the Preliminary Training School for general nurses.

1964   Physiotherapy clinic opened at Health Centre in Haverhill in November. A start was being made to implement the work study on the hospital domestic services.

1965   Mr. J. Burton appointed Hospital Catering Officer in April and Miss M. Finegan appointed Matron in June. Original pig sty demolished and car park provided in "B" Block. Work study on the domestic services being implemented including private contract for window and wall washing. Mr. T. H. Todd appointed as the first Domestic Supervisor. Exning Isolation Hospital sold. The first local "Back to Nursing" campaign held and the assistant cook training scheme introduced.

1966   The new Area laundry at Fulbourn Hospital opened and the laundry at Newmarket General Hospital closed.

1967   The South West (No. 1) Group HMC was disbanded. Newmarket General Hospital became part of the West Suffolk Group HMC at Bury St. Edmunds. "A" Block kitchen was converted to a changing room for ancillary staff. Mr. R. W. Heasman appointed Hospital Secretary. Mrs. E . Mason, Assistant Group Catering Officer retired. The mother and child unit opened in the childrens' ward C3 in June. Work started on upgrading the main theatres. The first Hospital Joint Consultative Committee formed in August. Mr. J. V. Burton appointed Catering Officer for the West Suffolk HMC and Miss Jenkins succeeded him as Hospital Catering Officer. Sewing room moved into new premises in the new central linen store.

1968   The Group Supplies Department moved from Ward B5 to new premises at Fulbourn Hospital. Ward C5 opened as mixed sex ophthalmic ward. Mr. J. Pountain, Hospital Dentist, resigned in October and 23 Field Terrace Road was purchased by the Ministry of Health to accommodate medical staff. A central topping-up linen and general stores service was introduced for wards and departments. Mr. W. Long the Head Porter, resigned. A start was made to introduce the new BBC 2 television programmes to the wards. Central dish wash up unit installed in "C" Block. Hospital laundry service transferred from Fulbourn Hospital to the new Area laundry at the West Suffolk Hospital in Bury St. Edmunds. Improved sluicing arrangements in the maternity unit opened.

1969   Work completed on upgrading the main theatres, which were opened in January. Ward B5 opened as female geriatric ward in June and a nurses' assisted transport service to and from Haverhill started. Ward C4 opened as a mixed sex professorial surgical ward. Liver transplant operation performed by Professor R. Calne at Newmarket General Hospital on 8th April. "Pay as you eat" service introduced for all staff in the staff restaurant in October. Mrs. V. Ranner, Sewing Room Superintendent for past 27 years retired. The General Nursing Council recommended permanent approval be given as a Training School for the Roll. Miss M. Finegan, Matron, retired in December. She was succeeded by Miss M. Armstrong as Senior Nursing Officer. Mrs. L. Macklin appointed Night Superintendent in October. The hospital Christmas arrangements changed.

1970   The original tramp wards and war time decontamination centre demolished and the entrance to the hospital improved. "A" ward above the maternity unit opened as a staff sick bay. In March a start was made to introduce a central sterile supply service to the wards and departments. Dr. I. P. Williams, Consultant Radiologist, resigned in July and Dr. A. W. Robertson, Consultant Anaesthetist and part-time Medical Superintendent retired in November. Three nursing staff posts were upgraded to Nursing Officers in line with the Salmon report in November.

1971 In March, Miss Jenkins, Hospital Catering Officer retired, succeeded by Mr. E. H. Eyre and Mr. A. J. Scotcher was appointed the first Voluntary Organiser. A meal vending machine installed in the staff restaurant, mainly for night staff meals. The Hospital League of Friends was formed in July and the first Hospital Awards Day was held in October. The new recovery/intensive care unit attached to main theatres opened in November. The staff health centre opened: Dr. J. M. Platts appointed Staff Health Officer.

1972 In April the Regional Hospital Board installed a standby electric generator which would meet all the needs of the hospital in the event of a breakdown in the electric power supply. The new day centre in "B" Block was opened by Mr. G. Gibson on 31st March. Building work started on the new nursery and ancillary rooms extension to the maternity unit. The ophthalmic unit in ward C5 moved to new premises at Addenbrooke's Hospital. Ward B5 closed. A small terrace house, 60 Exning Road, purchased by the Ministry of Health to accommodate nursing staff. Work study commenced on the hospital catering service in December. Another house, 89 St. Phillips Road, purchased by the Ministry of Health to accommodate nursing staff. Miss M. Armstrong, Senior Nursing Officer, resigned in December. Mr. W. S. Green appointed Fire Officer in April. A forty hour working week was introduced for all nursing staff in January.

1973 New nursery extension to maternity unit opened in March, coronary care unit opened in part of ward B2 in April and a patients' mechanical documentation system introduced in July.

1974 Dr. C. P. Hay, Consultant Chest Physician and Mr. E. S. Jamieson, Consultant Orthopaedic Surgeon, retired in February. The original porter's lodge and receiving rooms adjoining Exning Road demolished. Miss S. M. Stevens, Superintendent Physiotherapist, retired in June, being succeeded by Miss Hodge. The Hospital House Committee was abolished in March and the National Health Service was reorganised in April to contain both primary and secondary care. A form of line management was introduced. The hospital social work transferred to the Social Services Department, day to day administration of the health clinics at Newmarket and Mildenhall taken over by the hospital. A contractor specialised cleaning service started in the main kitchens. The West Suffolk Hospital (Best Buy) at Bury St. Edmunds opened.

1975 Administrative control of the hospital pathology laboratory transferred to Cambridge Health District (Teaching) in February. An Area Joint Consultative Staff Committee scheme was introduced. 75 and 23 Field Terrace Road and 60 Exning Road were sold.

1976 Opening hours for the Accident and Emergency Department restricted to 9 a.m. to 5.30 p.m. Monday to Friday. C.S.S.D. sterile pack system extended to local general practitioner surgeries.

1977 The new Post Graduate Medical Education Centre and Staff Recreation Room (the Gibson Centre) opened. Mr. R. W. Heasman, Unit Administrator, retired in May. Mr. G. Newbury, BA, appointed Unit Administrator in August.

1978 A new telephone exchange in "A" Block opened in June.

1979 Regional Health Authority agreed plans to upgrade and extend Wards B4 and B6 and in October approved the development of the Regional Rheumatology Unit at Newmarket General Hospital. The opening target date was set at April 1980. Ward C5 opened in March as Rheumatology unit. General practitioners given open access to physiotherapy department services.

1980 Ward C3 opened as a female surgical ward run on a 7 day basis. Dr. J. H. Dean, Consultant Pathologist, retired in June. Mr. F. Rich, District Administrator, retired in October and the Accident and Emergency department closed in November.

1981 Local general practitioners were given open access to the occupational therapy services at the hospital.

1982 The National Health Service was restructured from 1st April and the

Area Health Authority was abolished, being replaced by the West Suffolk Health Authority, based in Bury St. Edmunds. Mr. M. D. Corke, was Chairman and Mr. J. R, Melleney was District Administrator. In April the Department of Health and Social Security agreed that Newmarket General Hospital be designated a Demonstration Centre in Medical Rehabilitation (Rheumatology). Dr. J. M. Platts retired.

In the autumn of 1982 it was agreed necessary to totally rebuild Newmarket General Hospital because of its poor structural condition.

INDEX

Accident & Emergency Service 134, 135, 137, 138, 143, 144, 156, 183
"Achieving a Balance" 175, 176, 178, 179
Addenbrooke's Hospital 9, 10, 13, 21, 36, 76, 77, 78, 94, 95, 105, 107, 112, 113, 114, 119, 121, 130, 134, 135, 141, 143, 174, 182, 183, 184
Adlam, Mr. D. M. *(Consultant Oral Surgeon)* 162
Air Raid Precautions (A.R.P.) 49, 61, 75
Al Rafaie Dr. *(Consultant Pathologist)* 153
Albury, Major *(Group Military Registrar)* 65
Allard, Mr. *(Tramp)* 55
Allbert, Sir Clifford 37
Allen, Mrs. Stafford *(House Committee member)* 67
Allison, Mr. K.A.G. *(Hospital Engineer)* 80, 89, 107
Almoner/Medical Social Worker 106, 117, 133, 150, 156
Alper, Mr. S. 129
Ambulance Services 10, 16, 17, 83, 144, 161
Amdrus, Mrs. J. *(Voluntary Services Organiser)* 129
Annual Hospital Ball 103
Area Administrator 117, 134
Area Health Authorities 18, 19, 145
Area Medical Advisory Committee 18
Area Officers 18
Armed Forces 18
Armstrong, Miss. K. *(Senior Nursing Officer)* 126
Armstrong, Miss. M. *(Senior Nursing Officer)* 111, 124, 130
Arnott, Dr. J. *(Medical Staff)* 62
Ashman, Miss. *(Telephonist)* 65
Assistant Clerk & Steward 8
Assistant Hospital Secretary 8
Assisted Ventilation Unit 151, 153, 166
Atkinson, Mrs. Alice *(Ward Sister)* 110

Badge, Newmarket Hospital 87, 102
Bailey, Dr. Simon *(General Practitioner)* 175
Bakers Row 25, 49
Bannon, Dr. Roy *(Consultant Radiologist)* 154
Barling, Mrs. G. B. *(House Committee member)* 119
Barling, Nurse Natalie 67
Barnard, Mr. David *(Health Authority member)* 179
Barnard-Smith, Mr. *(Laundry)* 90
Barton, Mrs. D. *(Cook)* 91
Bartram, Mrs. *(Head Cook)* 91
Bastin, Mr. *(Operating Theatre)* 111, 122, 127
Beaty, Major 61, 62, 71
Bedlow, Mr. George *(Cook)* 38
Beeby, Mr. *(Cook)* 91
Bell, Mrs. I. *(Almoner)* 117, 133, 150
Beningfield, Charlotte *(Pauper)* 30
Benson, Mrs. *(Red X Library)* 68
Bentinck, Mrs. M. *(Linen Room Supervisor)* 149
Berridge, Dr. F. R. *(Consultant Radiologist)* 62
Berridge, Mrs. V. *(Radiographer)* 62

Berrigan, Mrs. Jean *(Senior Sister)*151
Blackburn, Mr. *(Deputy Clerk)* 37
Blackiston, Dr. *(Consultant Anaesthetist)* 88
Black Notley Hospital, Colchester 72
Blakey, Miss S. *(Dietitian)* 149
Blood Transfusion Centre 101
Board of Governors 10, 16
Board of Guardians 13, 14, 22, 25, 35, 37, 53, 88, 167, 170
Board Room 25, 123, 146
Boiler Capacity 45, 72
Boiler House 67, 105
Bonham, Mr. Boosh 37
Bonnin, Mr. Jasper Grant *(Orthopaedic Surgeon)* 65, 66, 71
Bowcock, Mr. *(Board of Guardians)* 37
Bowyer, Miss L. E. *(Senior Nursing posts)* 110, 111, 146, 149, 150, 153
Bratherton, Dr. D. *(Consultant Radiotherapist)* 153
Briggs Report 110
Bright, Mr. M. V. *(Consultant Obstetrician & Gynaecologist)* 139, 146, 150, 152, 163, 165, 166, 175
Brisco, Sister *(Out-patients)* 110
British Medical Association 16, 17
British Red Cross Society 15, 63, 86, 102, 129, 158
Brown, Miss *(Asst. Matron)* 111
Brown, Mr. Tom *(Town Clerk)* 58
"Brumey" *(Stoker)* 45
Brunel Health Service Organisation Unit 17
Bryson, Miss Kirsteen *(Senior Dietitian)* 159
Buck, Mr. H. R. OBE, JP. *(House Committee member)* 77, 94, 119
Bull, Mr. Eric *(Unit General Manager)* 152, 153, 155, 161, 165
Bullman, Mr. E. W. *(House Committee member)* 119
Burdon, Mr. G. H. *(Dispenser)* 63
Burton, Mr. B. A. *(General Administrator)* 152
Burton, Mr. J. *(Catering Officer)* 112, 118
Butler, Lady 63
Butler, Miss *(Sister Tutor)* 85
Butler, Mr. *(Senior Medical Staff)* 76
Butterfield, Sir John OBE, MD, FRCP *(Regius Professor of Physic)* 142
Bury St. Edmunds Health District 133, 141, 143, 145

Caesarea 11
Cairns, Mr. John *(Consultant Ophthalmic Surgeon)* 119, 130
Calne, Professor Sir Roy *(Consultant General Surgeon)* 121-123, 152
Calvert, Dr. John *(General Practitioner)* 175
Cambridge Chest Clinic 84
Cambridge, HRH The Duke of 168, 170
Cambridge Health District (Teaching) 134, 135, 145
Cambridgeshire County Council 9
Cardigan Street Nursing Home 22, 84, 95
Carter, Mr. Gordon *(Clerk)* 64
Casual Wards 49-52, 123
Casualties of War 14, 58, 59, 61, 63, 66, 67, 70, 72, 73, 74, 99

Catering Services 42-44, 56, 68, 73, 88, 90-92, 97, 101, 104, 106, 108, 112, 113, 118-120, 124, 127, 128, 130, 131, 133, 135, 142, 154, 159, 160
Catton, Canon Cedric *(Hospital Chaplain)* 171, 172
Caunt, Mr. *(Charge Nurse)* 111
Challice, Miss *(Typist)* 84, 94
Challise Close, Saxon Street 128
Chappell, Mr. *(Catering Advisor)* 99
Charlemagne 11
Chase Farm Hospital 7
Chase Farm Poor Law Schools 7
Cherry Cottages 25
"Cherry Tree" Public House 44, 50, 56, 74
Childrens' Ward 66
Chiropody 97, 157
Church *(Hospital Chapel)* 4, 49, 88, 108, 157, 167-172
Church Subscribers 167-168
Christmas arrangements 124, 154
Clark, Mr. R. F. A. *(House Committee member)* 119
Claydon, Sister *(Ward Sister)* 111, 149
Cleghorn, Miss *(Home Sister)* 111
Clerk to the Guardians 25, 29, 37
Cleveland House 66, 70, 77
Cockleton, Miss Jessie *(Dining Room Assistant)* 123
Coleman, Mr. Fred 50, 74
Community Health Council 18, 174, 179, 182
Community Hospital 176, 180-185
Concerts 68
Confidential Enquiry into Peri-operative deaths (CEPOD) 175, 176, 178, 179
Coni, Dr. Nick *(Consultant Geriatrician)* 134, 152
Constant, Mr. Chris *(Consultant Orthopaedic Surgeon)* 159
Convalescent Hospitals (see Home Place)
Cooke, Mr. Peter M. *(Group Secretary/Area Administrator)* 117, 134
Cooper, Miss Julie *(Patsat Implementation Officer)* 161
Cooper, Dr. Pamela *(Consultant Pathologist)* 152
Cooper, Paul & Associates 179
Copeman, Mr. *(Gardener)* 92, 104
Copthorne Hospital 112
Corke, Mr. Martin D. *(Chairman)* 117, 166, 179
Coster, Mr. J. B. *(Chairman)* 67, 77
Coston, Mr. *(Tramp)* 55
Cowper-Johnson, Miss *(Superintendent Radiographer)* 93, 100, 144
Crease, Mr. John *(County Architect)* 53
Crisp, Dr. Adrian *(Consultant Rheumatologist)* 154
Croft Road 165
Crompton, Dr. *(Medical Staff)* 36
Central Sterile Supply Department (CSSD) 125, 137
Cudden, Sister *(Ward Sister)* 91, 110
Culank, Dr. Les *(Consultant Pathologist)* 151, 152
Cullen, Miss D. *(Radiographer)* 62
Curtis, Mrs. *(Laundry Superintendent)* 90, 92

Dandy, Mr. David *(Consultant Orthopaedic Surgeon)* 131, 141, 150, 152, 155, 166
Darling, Miss Diana *(Nurse)* 67
Darval, Mrs. I. *(Telephonist)* 86
Davison, Dr. William *(Consultant Geriatrician)* 106, 121
Day, Mr. H. *(League of Friends)* 128, 135
Day Surgery 141, 161, 162, 175, 183, 184
Dean, Dr. John H. *(Consultant Pathologist)* 93, 100, 103, 142, 153
Deasley, Mr. *(Painter)* 86
Dennis, Rt. Rev. John *(Bishop St. Edmundsbury & Ipswich)* 172
Dental Surgery 71, 101
Department of Health 17, 57, 138, 175, 182, 183, 185 (see also Ministry of Health)
Deputy Hospital Secretary 8
Deputy House Governor 5
Derby, Lord 93
Diet 27, 28, 29,
Dingle, Mr. J. T. D.Sc. Ph.D. *(Strangeways Director)* 142
Dispensary *(Infirmary)* 36
District Administrator 5, 133, 134, 143, 146
District General Manager 5, 145, 150, 154, 163, 165, 171, 175, 179, 182, 183
District Health Authorities 145
District Management Board 154, 179
District Management Team 18, 133-136, 139, 142, 144-146, 173
District Medical Committee 18, 141, 179
Domestic Superintendent 108
Dorrell, Mr. Stephen MP *(Parliamentary Under Secretary of State)* 183
Drake, Miss D. *(Medical Records)* 130, 145
Dunachie, Miss Ann *(Nurse Manager)* 11, 153, 155, 156, 163, 165
Dunston, Miss *(Physiotherapist)* 115

East Anglian Regional Health Authority 133, 136-138, 141, 142, 145, 151, 162, 173-175, 178-180, 182-184
East Anglian Thoracic Medicine Advisory Committee 151
Easter, Mr. Herbert *(Chargehand Porter)* 38
East Suffolk Health Authority 166, 185
Ebford 8
Edmundson, Canon E. 108, 172
Edward VII, HRH King 170
Elliot, Mr. Grant *(Director of Finance and Information)* 179
Ellis, Dr. Shirley *(Area Pharmaceutical Officer)* 138
Ely, The Rt. Rev. The Lord Bishop of 167, 168
Emergency Services Hospitals 9, 14, 15, 54, 58, 59-81
Enfield Poor Law Institution 7
English, Mr. *(Kitchen Porter)* 43
English National Board 153, 159, 163
Ennion, Major S. J. *(Clerk to Board of Govenors)* 37, 53
Environmental Health Service 18
Essex House 25, 27
Evans, Dr. I. *(Consultant Physician)* 139
Evans, Mrs. Pamela *(Clinical Nurse Manager)* 163
Ewan, Dr. I. B. *(Regional Medical Officer)* 83, 126
Executive Councils 16

Exeter 8
Exeter Acute Hospitals 8
Exmouth Community Mental Handicap Services 8
Exning Cricket Club 8
Exning Isolation Hospital 21, 84, 94, 95, 113
Exning Road 25, 44, 47, 49, 130, 136
Exning Road Working Mens' Club 49
Eyre, Mr. E. H. *(Catering Officer)* 128, 149, 159

Fairbairn, Mrs. J. *(Head Occupational Therapist)* 152
Fairlay, Mrs. A. *(Personnel Manager)* 165
Family Planning 17, 103
Family Practitioner Committee 18
Farahty, Sister *(Ward Sister)* 111
Field Terrace 25, 119, 131, 136
Finch, Miss R. E. *(Matron)* 78, 81, 93, 110
Finegan, Miss *(Matron)* 110, 111, 112, 124
Fire Services 10, 86, 126, 135
Fisher, Miss P. *(Clerk)* 64
Flack, Mr. Eric *(Health Authority member)* 179
Ford, Miss *(Assistant Matron)* 111
Foster, Miss *(Matron, Exning Isolation Hospital)* 95
Foulden Terrace 25
Fountain, Mr. J. *(Hospital Dentist)* 120
Freeman, Miss D. *(Telephonist)* 86
Fulbourn 22, 84, 90, 97, 102, 115, 118, 120, 141
Funeral Arrangements 37
Fussell, Lt. Col. Ruth *(USAF Nursing Officer)* 118

Gairdner, Dr. Douglas *(Consultant Paediatrician)* 107
Gallon, Mr. Jimmy *(Workhouse Inmate)* 37
Gardener, The Rev. *(Chaplain)* 69, 172
Garmory, Mr. J. S. *(Clerk)* 71, 145
General Managers 19
General Nursing Council 57, 70, 78, 98, 102, 115, 117, 119, 124 (see also English National Board)
General Practitioners 16, 17, 36, 53, 54, 76, 95, 133, 134, 137, 139, 142, 143, 144, 156, 158, 175, 176, 183, 184, 185
Geriatric 21, 36, 105, 106, 113, 114, 120, 121, 125, 129, 131, 134, 141, 143, 157, 174, 175
German Prisoners of War 73, 74, 79
Gibbons, Miss *(Home Sister)* 64
Gibson, Mr. A. S. C. JP 119, 142, 162, 186
Gibson Centre 138, 139, 155, 176
Gibson, Mr. G. S. 10, 129
Gilbert Act 1782 13, 21, 49
Gill, Dr. Morton *(Medical Staff)* 65, 66
Glanz, Mrs. S. *(Nursing Manager)* 156
Goble, Mr. Dennis *(District Nursing Officer)* 159
Goodchild, Miss E. M. *(Clerk)* 71
Gould, Mr. Peter *(Clerk)* 64
Grace, Mr. *(Tramp)* 51

Grange Maternity Home, Ely 84
Gray, Dr. Clement *(Medical Staff)* 36
Gray, Dr. Gilbert *(Medical Staff)* 36
Gray, Dr. Norman *(Medical Staff)* 36, 128
Green, Mr. Dunstal *(Workhouse Inmate)* 45
Green, Mr. W. S. *(Group Fire Officer)* 130, 137
Greenwich District Hospital 7
Gregg, Dr. Duncan *(Consultant Radiologist)* 89, 93
Grey Book *(Reorganisation 1974)* 19, 133
Griffiths, Mr. Eldon MP 138, 162, 176, 178, 180, 183
Griffiths Report *(NHS Management Inquiry)* 19, 154
Group Medical Advisory Committee 93
Grundy, Mrs. Lois *(District Catering Manager)* 160
Guillebaud Report 96
Gurteen, Mr. *(Board of Guardians member)* 37
Guy, Mr. Charles *(Workhouse Master)* 38
Gwynne Terrace 25

Haigh, Sister *(Ward Sister)* 153
Hamilton, Rev. Douglas *(Hospital Chaplain)* 172
Hammond, Mr. P. 78, 104
Hardy, Mrs. Sheila *(Asst. Domestic Services Manager)* 149, 154
Harvey, Miss E. J. *(Superintendent Physiotherapist)* 146, 151
Harvey, Mr. *(Foreman Gardener)* 40, 41
Haslam, Mrs. J. *(Medical Records Officer)* 146, 151
Hatcher, Dr. *(Consultant Radiologist)* 139, 143, 152, 154, 156
Hatley, Mr. W. B. *(Relieving Officer)* 51, 54
Hawes, Dr. *(Medical Staff)* 75, 80
Hawkins, Major Bailey *(Transport Officer)* 73, 74
Hawkins, Mr. *(Assistant Sanitary Inspector)* 58
Hawkins, Rev. R. *(Hospital Chaplain)* 172
Hay, Dr. C. P. *(Medical Staff)* 131
Hay, Miss S. M. *(Matron)* 93, 97, 100, 110
Hayter, Miss *(Physiotherapist)* 71, 93
Haytor, Miss V. *(Masseuse)* 63
Hayward, Sister *(Ward Sister)* 110, 128
Hazard, Mr. Bill *(Head Gardener)* 114
Hazleton, Mr. *(Internal Auditor)* 53
Hazleman, Dr. Brian *(Consultant Rheumatologist)* 149, 152, 154, 166
Health Centres 17, 83
Health Districts 19
Health Visiting 17
Heasman, Mrs. Ada V. 7, 8, 54, 66, 110
Heasman, Mr. Ernest S. 7, 8, 54, 59, 66, 83, 85, 145
Heasman Family 4, 7, 8
Heasman, George R. L. 4, 8, 51, 58
Heasman, John R. 8
Heasman, Michael S. 8
Heasman, Richard W. 4, 6, 7, 8, 115, 139, 145, 173
Heasman, Miss Rosanna R. 8
Heathfields House 70, 77

Heathside 69
Helicopters 115
Henry, Brigadier T. R. *(Group Secretary)* 83, 84, 85, 87
Hesketh, Mr. J. S. *(Consultant Obstetrician & Gynaecologist)* 95
Higgins, Mr. W. *(Unit Works Officer)* 162, 165
Hinchingbrooke Hospital, Huntingdon 140, 151, 174
Hinnel, Mr. *(Public Assistance Officer)* 53
Hipwell, Sister A. *(Theatre Sister)* 160
History of Hospitals 11-20 (chapter one)
Hobbs, Miss Ruth *(Assistant Nurse)* 63, 67
Hobbs, Mr. W. *(Pharmacist)* 89, 100, 102
Hodge, Miss G. *(Superintendent Physiotherapist)* 132, 149, 151
Hogan, Miss Melanie *(Catering Officer)* 159, 160
Hollands, Messrs. *(Contractors)* 71
Holtz, Mr. H. *(Superintendent Engineer)* 106
Home Nursing and Midwifery 17, 83
Home Place Convalescent Home 153
Honours and Awards:
    Penney, Miss A. 145, 150
    Dandy, Mr. D. 150
    Tagart, Mr. R. E. B. 153
    Maycock, Mr. Leo 155
Hospital Advisory Service 131, 155
Hospital Chaplains 123, 167-173
Hospital Management Committees: 16, 17
    South West (No.1) 9, 16, 83, 97, 115, 118
    West Suffolk 10, 115, 117, 125, 128
Hospital Medical Staff Committee 86, 91, 99, 126, 140, 146, 149, 151, 154, 155, 162, 166, 178, 179, 180, 183
Hospital Open Days 75, 87, 155, 161
Hospital Secretary 5, 7, 8, 111, 115, 126, 133, 135 (see also Unit Administrator)
Houghton, Mrs. L. *(Personnel Officer)* 162
House Committees 16, 53, 67, 73, 74, 77, 112, 117-119, 128, 129, 132
Hughes, Taffy *(Finance Staff)* 88
Hulme, Mr. Arthur *(Regional Work Study)* 108
Humphries, Mr. *(Chimney Sweep)* 63, 75
Hunt, Mr. W. H. *(House Committee member)* 67
Huntingdon County Hospital 84
Hurst, Geoff *(Regional Admin. Staff)* 83
Hutchby, Dr. J. P. *(Consultant in Public Health Medicine)* 175
Hydrotherapy 93, 125, 140

Industrial Action 127, 131, 134-138, 140, 141, 160
Infectious Diseases Hospitals 15, 21
Infirmary 9, 14, 35-48
Institute of Health Service Administrators 7
Ipswich Health District 133
Ipswich Hospital 113

Jacobs, Mr. 41
Jacobs, Mrs. O. *(Nursing Officer)* 150

Jamieson, Mr. E. S. *(Consultant Surgeon)* 71, 75, 76, 80, 87, 93, 112, 121, 131
Jarvis, Vivian *(Nursing Staff)* 67, 86
Jenkins, Mrs. *(Catering Officer)* 118, 127
Jockey Association of Great Britain 125
Johnson, Mr. Brian *(Administrator)* 151, 155, 160
Joint Consultative Committee 18, 118, 134, 136
Jones, Miss A. *(Nursing Officer)* 150
Jones, Dr. Arden *(Medical Staff)* 62, 66, 68, 77, 130, 137
Jones, Mr. Graham *(prospective MP)* 142
Jones, Mr. Robert H. *(Unit General Manager)* 165
Jubb, Dr. R. *(Consultant Rheumatologist)* 152

Kallend, Mrs. A. *(Dietitian)* 159
Kaye brothers *(Porters)* 57
Kelly, Air Vice Marshal *(Medical Superintendent)* 80, 93
Kemp-Turner, Mr. Kenneth 179, 181, 182
Kendall, Mr. N. E. *(Asst. Master etc)* 57, 83
Kennedy, Mr. Colin *(Consultant Urologist)* 155
Kent, Mr. A. S. *(Chairman)* 118, 119
Kerridge Ltd. *(Contractors)* 129
Kerrigan, Dr. G. N. W. *(Consultant Physician)* 139, 146, 150, 152, 166
Kerslake, Mrs. *(Pharmacy)* 92
King, Capt. H. R. CBE JP. *(House Committee)* 53, 73, 128
King, Mr. Jim *(Inmate)* 41
King Edward VII Hospital, Windsor 8
King Edward Road 25
Kings of Exning *(Contractors)* 65
Kingston House Rooms, Newmarket 22, 25
Kingswell, Sister *(Theatre Sister)* 60, 111
Kirk, Miss B. R. *(Pathology Manager)* 165
Knox, Mr. J. S. *(District Domestic Manager)* 136

Lamb, Mr. Robert *(Consultant Ophthalmologist)* 150, 152
Lambert, Miss Ethel *(Laundress)* 57
Lambert, Miss Violet *(Asst. Matron)* 57, 63
Langley, Mr. A. F. *(Manager, Temperance Hotel)* 61
Large, Mrs. Sonia *(Deputy Medical Records Officer)* 160
Laundry and Linen Services 41, 42, 56, 65, 67, 72, 74, 89, 90, 102, 106, 113, 115, 118-120, 136, 154
Lawrence, Miss D. *(Clerk to Medical Superintendent)* 62
Leader & Griffiths *(Funeral Directors)* 37
Leader, Doreen *(Nursing Staff)* 67
League of Friends 10, 97, 128, 136, 145, 153, 159, 160, 161, 163
Lee, Mrs. E. *(Superintendent Radiographer)* 149
Leicester 8
Lester, Mr. P. *(Catering Manager)* 161
Leys School, Cambridge 76
Lincoln 8
Lindrum, Mr. *(Victoria Hotel/Cinema)* 48
Linton Close 113
Lions Club 10

Lithgow, Miss *(Matron)* 60, 78, 110
Little Plumstead Hospital 84
Livock, Mrs. Ada Violet 7, 8
Livock, Mr. Edward 7
Livock, Mr. William 7
Local Health Authorities 14, 16, 133
Lockhead, Mr. *(Tailor)* 45
Lockhead, Georgina H. *(Assistant Nurse)* 38
Lomas, Mary *(Nursing Staff)* 67
Long, Mr. W. *(Head Porter)* 119
"Lovejoy" 154
Lum, Dr. C. *(Consultant Chest Physician)* 135, 140-142
Lyimo, Miss A. *(Theatre Nursing Officer)* 150
Lycett-Green, Sir Stephen *(RHB Chairman)* 104
Lyles, Staff Nurse 111
Lyons, Messrs. J. 90, 91, 99

MacCracken, Dr. *(County Medical Officer of Health)* 53
McBrien, Mr. Michael *(Consultant General Surgeon)* 152
McKenna, The Hon. Mrs. E. *(House Committee member)* 119
McKinsey 17
McLeod, Sister V. 151
Macklin, Mrs. *(Night Superintendent)* 111, 124
Maher, Dr. E. A. *(Anaesthetist)* 152
Malachi, Rev. H. A. P. *(Hospital Chaplain)* 108, 172
Market Street 61
Marrlott, Miss *(First Aid Post)* 64
Marshall, Mr. Sid *(RDC Staff)* 58
Martin. Miss M. M. R. *(Consultant Obstetrician & Gynaecologist)* 152
Mason, Mrs. E. *(Kitchen Superintendent)* 90, 91, 117
Mason, Mr. H. *(Head Gardener)* 149
Master *(Workhouse)* 38, 53, 54, 57-59, 64, 83, 145
Maternity 22, 35, 36, 67, 68, 69, 83, 88, 95, 97, 105, 107, 114, 115, 117, 120, 126, 127, 128, 130, 139, 141, 150, 152, 153, 157, 161, 163, 164, 174, 183, 184
Matron 7, 36, 37, 53, 54, 58, 60, 66, 78, 80, 81, 97, 100, 110, 111, 121, 124
Maund, Dr. *(Medical Staff)* 36
Maxwell, Professor *(Medical Staff)* 62, 85
Maycock, Mr. Leo *(Theatre Staff)* 86, 111, 155
Meadowcroft, Mr. G. *(Group Treasurer)* 83, 88, 115
Medical Records 86, 87, 99, 109, 112, 114, 129-131, 142, 146, 151, 160
Medical Officer *(Workhouse)* 28, 29, 31
Melton Asylum 22, 44
Melleney, Mr. John R. *(Chief Executive)* 4, 146, 175, 179
Meredith, Miss *(Sister Tutor)* 85, 111
Merrin, Mr. H. *(Group Engineer)* 83, 106
Mid Anglia Community Health NHS Trust 4, 185
Midgley-Revett, Mrs. *(Medical Records Officer)* 149
Mildenhall Workhouse 22
Miles, Sister (Outpatient Sister) 160
Military Hospitals 15, 23
Milne, Mr. Fred *(Night Telephonist)* 86, 109, 123

Mingay, Mr. Bert *(RDC Staff)* 58
Ministry of Health 58, 59, 60, 62, 65-66, 71, 72, 75-77, 80, 85, 92, 98, 99, 101, 105, 107, 113-115, 119, 127, 130 (see also Department of Health)
Ministry of Pension Hospitals 15
Minter, Mr. Vic *(RHB Administration)* 83
Minter, Mr. Vincer *(Master)* 37, 169
Minter, Mrs. Alice Vincer *(Matron)* 37, 110, 170
Mitchell, Mr. C. *(Group Secretary)* 84
Moffat, Mr. David *(Consultant ENT Surgeon)* 152
Moleneux, Mr. *(Tramp)* 55
Monkton, Mr. *(Consultant Ophthalmologist)* 150
Morrey, Dr. *(Consultant Pathologist)* 93
Mortuary 37, 65, 68, 97
Mowl, Miss D. *(Telephonist)* 86
Multitone Pocket Paging 100
Munsey, Mr. *(County Council Clerk)* 53
Murray, Mrs. A. T. *(Acting Matron)* 121
Murray, Dr. *(Pathologist)* 65

Nash, Miss *(Typist)* 84
National Federation of Building Trade Operatives 76
National Health Service 4, 9, 14-16, 57, 70
NHS & Community Care Act 1990 179, 180, 181
Neville, Mr. S. N. 125
Newbury, Mr. Geoffrey *(Unit Administrator)* 139, 146, 149, 150, 152
New Chesterton Window Cleaning Co. Ltd. 113
Newman, Mrs. B. *(Night Nursing Officer)* 160, 165
Newmarket Journal Xmas Fund 10, 87, 99, 102, 108, 120, 131, 142, 153, 160, 161, 165
Newmarket Lawn Tennis Club 71
Newmarket Poor Law Institution 7, 8
Newmarket Urban/Rural District Council 58, 88, 97, 102, 106, 125, 128
Newmarket Town Band 56, 87
Newstead, Mrs. Moira *(Clinical Manager)* 163
Newton, Mr. Bertie *(Board of Guardians/House Committee)* 37, 53, 67, 73
Nicol, Mr. Duncan CBE, MA, AHSM. (NHS Management Executive) 163
Night Superintendent *(Office)* 36, 111
Norfolk Cottage 25
Norfolk, Duchess of 165
Norfolk & Norwich Hospital 67
North, Mr. A. K.*(Deputy Administrator)* 149, 151
Northampton General Hospital 13
Nottingham City Hospital 7
Nurse Training School 38, 70, 78, 85, 87, 98, 102, 106, 111, 117-119, 123, 124, 143, 153, 156, 159, 162, 163

Oakfield House 73, 77, 100, 101, 104, 113
O'Callaghan, Mrs. *(Red Cross)* 87, 119, 129
Occupational Health Service 18, 157
Occupational Therapy/Remedial Medicine Dept. 67, 96, 113, 114, 144, 152, 157, 159
Operating Theatres 75, 93, 95, 111, 114, 118, 120, 122, 123, 126, 129, 144, 150, 153, 155-157, 159, 160, 175

Ophthalmic 119, 130, 157
Order of St. John of Jerusalem 15
Osborne House 73
O'Sullivan, Mrs. Patricia *(Asst. General Manager)* 163
Otterspoor, Gladys 31
Outdoor Relief 53, 54

Page, Mr. Frank *(Asst. Master)* 57
Paice, Mr. James MP 176
Papworth Hospital 101, 126, 142, 151, 166
Parkers Garage 75
Parkinson, Mr. V. R. *(P.T. Instructor)* 77
Parr, Sister D. *(Nurse Tutor)* 111, 145
Parton, Mrs. Jean *(Manager Midwifery)* 161
Patey, Dr. Geoffrey *(District Community Physician)* 135
Pathology 35, 65, 68, 75, 134, 135, 149, 155, 158, 159, 165
Patient Satisfaction Survey 126, 161
Pawsey, Mr. Gerald *(Unit Treasurer)* 165
Paxton Park Maternity Hospital 84
Pearce, Dr. A. J. *(Consultant Anaesthetist)* 152, 163, 165, 166
Pearmain, Mr. *(Relieving Officer)* 54
Pearmain, Mr. G. S. *(Deputy Group Secretary)* 84
Pearmain, Nurse 83
Peck, Miss (Staff) 63
Penney, Miss A. *(Senior Nursing Officer)* 111, 145, 150
Personal Social Services 18
Peterborough 8
Pharmacy 98, 102, 137, 138, 158
Pharaoh Ant 125, 126
Pharaoh, Mrs G. *(Deputy Nursing Manager)* 156, 160, 162
Phillips, Mr. Anthony *(Pharmacy Services Manager)* 163
Physiotherapy 55, 64, 71, 75, 87, 93-95, 108, 114, 115, 117, 125, 130, 142, 144, 158, 159
Platt Report 110
Platt, Sir Harry 110
Platts, Dr. J. M. *(House Physician)* 30, 66, 68, 129, 145
Plymouth 8
Poliomyelitis 71, 80, 94, 99, 105
Poor Law Commission 25, 27, 28, 29, 31
Poor Law Infirmaries 35-48
Poor Law Legislation 12, 13, 14, 27, 28, 29, 35, 53
Porritt Report 17
Post-Graduate Medical Centre 135, 137, 156
Prigg *(Family Butchers)* 44
Primrose Lane Maternity Hospital 84
Princess of Wales RAF Hospital 163
Prison Health Service 18
Pritchard, Mr. Robert *(Porter)* 57
Prizegiving, Nurses 85, 88, 93, 98, 106, 118, 126, 129, 153, 159, 160, 162, 163, 165, 166
Prospect Terrace 25
Pryor, Sister *(Ward Sister)* 159

Public Assistance Institutions:
   Epping 8
   Leicester 8
   Lincoln 8
   Newmarket 8, 9, 53-60, 66
   Sudbury 8, 62
   Watford 8
   York 8
Pudney Cup 88
Pulvertaft, Dr. Roger *(Consultant Radiologist)* 156
Purser, Mrs. *(Staff Pharmacist)* 153
Pye, Dr. R. J. *(Consultant Dermatologist)* 152
Pym, Mr. Francis MC MP 106

Rae, Dr. *(Deputy County Medical Officer of Health)* 53
Rahill, Charge Nurse E. 57
Ramsey, Mrs. F. W. *(House Committee member)* 67, 77
Ranner, Mrs. V. *(Sewing Room Superintendent)* 124
Red Cross Library 68
Redevelopment 173-186 (see also Upgrading works)
Redfern, Mr. *(Gas Company)* 46
Regional Health Authorities 18, 173
Regional Hospital Board 16, 17, 83, 86, 90, 104, 105, 108, 109, 113-115, 120, 126, 127
Regional Medical Advisory Committee 18
Regional Officers 18, 83, 126
Relieving Officers 51, 53, 54
Retention of Newmarket General Hospital, Committee for 177-182
Reorganisation 9, 17, 19, 83, 133, 145, 179-181
Resuscitation Room 64
Rheumatology 140-143, 145, 149, 156, 184
Rich, Mr. F. R. *(District Administrator)* 134, 143, 151
Riddington, Mr. H. *(Engineer)* 44
Riversfield Sub-Normal Hospital 84
Roberton, Dr. N. *(Consultant Paediatrician)* 152
Robertson, Dr. A. W. *(Consultant Anaesthetist)* 91, 102, 123, 126
Robinson, Mr. Nigel *(Unit Management Accountant)* 146, 150, 155, 162, 165
Robinson, Sister *(Ward Sister)* 60
Roddy, Miss *(Nursing Officer)* 127
Rodman, Mr. *(Head Porter)* 92
Rogers, Dr. *(County Medical Officer of Health)* 53
Rolfe, Mr. *(Laundry Worker)* 90
Rolfe, Sister *(Theatre Sister)* 111
Rolles, Mr. Keith *(Consultant General Surgeon)* 152
Ronald, Mr. K. *(Night Telephonist)* 86, 109
Rotary Club of Newmarket 129, 130
Round Table:
   Newmarket 114, 117
   Bury St. Edmunds 92
Rous Memorial Hospital 21, 69
Rowe, Sister L. M. *(Night Superintendent)* 124
Rowlands, Mr. J. *(Consultant Surgeon)* 60, 62, 65, 71, 74, 78, 79, 92

Rowley, Sir Joshua *(Lord Lieutenant)* 155
Royal College of Nursing 110
Royal College of Surgeons 96, 162, 175, 178
Royal Corps of Signals 8
Royal Devon & Exeter Hospitals *(Heavitree)* 8
Royal Hospitals 13
Royston General Hospital 84
Royston Maternity Hospital 84
Rushton, Mr. Neil *(Consultant Orthopaedic Surgeon)* 152
Rutherford, Mrs Jane *(Director Planning & Personnel)* 180
Ryle, Professor *(Regius Professor)* 66

Saffron Walden General Hospital 84
St. Alphege's Hospital 7
St. Edmundsbury & Ipswich, Bishop of 88
St. Fabians' 78, 85, 94, 98, 100, 101,102, 104
St. James' Hospital 84
St. Marylebone Poor Law Institution 7
St. Mary's Hospital, Bury St. Edmunds 137
St. Michael's Hospital, Enfield 7
St. Peter's, York 11
St. Philips Church 169, 170, 172
St. Phillips Hall 69
St. Phillips Terrace 25
Salmon Report 110, 111, 127
Sarbutt, Miss *(Asst. Matron)* 78, 111
Sargent, Miss K. A. G. *(Deputy Superintendent Physiotherapist)* 93
Saunders, Miss A. *(Staff Pharmacist)* 149, 153
Sayers, Mrs Elizabeth *(Deputy Editor, Newmarket Journal)* 152
Sayers, Mr. *(County Council Accountant)* 53
School Health Services 16,17
Scotcher, Mr. A. J.*(Voluntary Services Organiser)* 128, 129
Scott, Canon C. *(Hospital Chaplain)* 172
Scott, Mr. P. M. *(Consultant Orthopaedic Surgeon)* 152
Seaman, Dr. Muriel *(Consultant Pathologist)* 152
Sectors 18
Sector Administrator 8
Senior Clerk 8
Security 47-48
Senior Nursing Officer 110, 111, 126
Shave, Mr. Christopher *(Pauper)* 30
Shepherd, Mrs. Gillian MP 176
Shepherd, Sister *(Ward Sister)* 60
Shneerson, Dr. John *(Consultant Physician)* 151-153, 155, 162, 166, 175
Sidcup 8
Siklos, Dr. Paul *(Consultant Physician)* 152
Simpson, Dr. Norman 36
Simpson & Sons *(Contractors)* 167
Sinclair, Miss M. *(Nursing Officer)* 127, 150
Skipp, Sister *(Ward Sister)* 111, 149
Skull, Mrs. Amanda *(Manager)* 165

Smellie, Mr. W. A. B. *(Consultant General Surgeon)* 175
Smith, Mrs. Lamport *(Almoner)* 117
Smith, Mr. Nigel *(Administrator)* 160
Smith, Mrs. Winnie *(Transplant Patient)* 122
Social Services 10, 18
South West (No.1) Group HMC 9, 10, 16, 83
Southwold 8
Spiller, Miss E. M. *(Sister Tutor)* 85
Staff, shortages of 75-77, 79, 81, 87, 96, 102, 107, 153, 160, 161, 163, 174, 182
Stamford Terrace 25
Starcross 8
Statistical Information:
    Bed numbers 54, 72, 94, 98, 105, 107, 123, 156, 165, 181
    Costs 69, 97, 98, 100, 103, 105
    Patients 61, 62, 67, 69, 72, 74, 75, 78, 90, 98, 103, 138, 139, 146, 151, 156, 164, 165, 181
    Staff 38, 62, 67, 77, 90, 129
Stead, Dr. B. R. *(Consultant Anaesthetist)* 152
Steel, Dr. Y. *(Consultant Radiologist)* 152
Steggles, Messrs. *(Contractors)* 25
Stevens, Miss S. M. *(Superintendent Physiotherapist)* 71, 93, 94, 132
Stone, Dr. David *(Consultant Cardiologist)* 160
Stradbroke, Rt. Hon. Earl of 98
Sudbury Poor Law Institution 7
Suffolk Area Health Authority 133, 134, 135, 141
Suffolk County Council 9
Suffolk Health Authority 166, 185
Summary of Services 1986 156
Sunlight Hospital Services 154
Swann, Miss B. *(Laundry Superintendent)* 67
Symonds, Mr. Fred *(Storesman)* 109

Tagart, Mr. R. E. B. *(Consultant General Surgeon)* 92, 146, 150, 152, 153
Tamlyn, Mrs. Susan *(Health Authority member)* 179
Taylor, Mr. J. G. *(Board of Guardians/House Committee member)* 37, 77
Taylor, Nurse Mary 67
Taylor, Miss Perris *(Consultant Ophthalmologist)* 119
Telephones 65, 86, 96, 101, 108, 109, 125, 138, 139, 140
Terry, Mr. Philip *(Staff Pharmacist)* 159
Thomas, Mr. Frank *(Asst. Master)* 57
Thompson, Mr. G. *(Pharmacist)* 67, 75
Thompson, Mrs. *(Masseuse)* 63
Thompson, Mr. Freddie *(Public Assistance Officer)* 53
Thompson, J.J & Partners *(Consultant Advisers)* 181, 182
Thorborne, Mr. *(Group Catering Officer)* 101
Three Counties Hospital, Bedford 67
Todd, Mr. T. H. *(Domestic Superintendent)* 113
Tomlin, Mr. *(Laundry)* 90
Tomlinson, Mr. Frank *(RDC Surveyor)* 58
Tower Hospital, Ely 84
Transplant Surgery 121-123

Trent, Mr. *(Local Baker)* 91
Troughton, Mr. *(Board of Guardians)* 37, 46
Tuberculosis patients 64, 66, 67, 71, 72, 77, 87, 92, 96, 97, 99, 105
Turner, Miss A. *(Nursing Officer)* 156
Turner, Mr. *(Lyons Catering Advisor)* 90, 91
Tyler, Nurse Heather 67

Unit Administrator 133, 134, 146
Unit General Manager 145, 150, 152, 153, 154, 155, 164
Unit Management Group 146, 150, 152, 154, 155, 159, 161, 162, 163, 165
Unit Matrons 127
University College Hospital 119
Union of Parish Houses 9, 14, 25 - 33
U. S. Military Hospital, Lakenheath 23, 118
Upgrading works 55, 90, 92, 94, 98-100, 103, 104, 106, 107, 113, 114, 118, 120, 121, 123, 127, 129, 130, 137, 139, 142, 147, 151, 152, 153, 155, 159
Upton Hospital, Slough 8

Vaccination and Immunisation 16, 17, 29, 129
Vagrancy Acts 12
Vaile, Rev. A. *(Hospital Chaplain)* 169, 172
Van den Brul, Dr. *(Anaesthetist)* 152
Van Woerden, Miss A. R. *(District Director of Midwifery Services)* 153
Varley, Mr. *(Porter and Gardener)* 21
Varley, Mr. E. W. B. *(Consultant Oral Surgeon)* 152, 162
Varley, Mrs. Rosie *(Health Authority member)* 179, 185
Victoria, HRH Queen 170
Victoria Villa 25
Vogel, Miss *(Assistant Nurse)* 63
Voluntary Hospitals 13, 14
Voluntary Services Organiser 120, 126, 128, 129, 158

Wales, HRH The Prince of 21, 168, 170, 172
Wales, HRH The Princess of 151, 163
Wallace, Sir Richard 21
Walnut Tree Hospital, Sudbury 7, 77, 84
Walsham-le-Willows 73
Wanless, Mr. James *(Tramp)* 51, 52
Warren, Dr. R. *(Consultant Pathologist)* 152
Wards:
        A1 - 78, 79, 88, 111
        A2 - 69, 74, 93, 95
        A3 - 65, 66, 77, 141
        B1 - 78, 125, 155, 159
        B2 - 72, 75, 111, 118, 125, 131, 144
        B3 - 76, 114, 138, 145
        B4 - 72, 77, 111, 140, 141, 143, 151, 153
        B5 - 65, 77, 118, 120, 138
        B6 - 65, 72, 77, 110, 129, 140, 141, 143
        C1 - 79
        C3 - 80, 107, 111, 114, 118, 142, 160, 162

C4 - 120, 121, 122, 159, 165
C5 - 78, 114, 119, 120, 121, 130, 140, 142,153
C6 - 76, 144
C7 - 78, 80, 88, 98, 113, 114, 144, 156
C8 - 91, 110, 111, 144, 160, 165
C9 - 110, 128, 144
Ward Blocks:
"A" - 42, 45, 48, 58, 61, 63-68, 70, 83, 90, 91, 95, 97, 98, 102, 107, 115, 128, 139, 140, 141, 147, 153
"B" - 61, 63, 64, 65, 67, 68, 70, 87, 95, 103, 106, 107, 111, 113, 114, 120, 129, 147, 150, 153, 173
"C" - 61, 65-68, 70, 75, 90, 91, 95, 98, 114, 117, 118, 120, 126, 127, 131, 135, 137, 141, 142, 147, 150, 173
Watford 8
Watsham, Dr. C. P. *(Anaesthetist)* 152
Watson, Colonel *(Medical Superintendent)* 60, 62, 75, 80, 93
Watson, Mr. John *(Consultant Ophthalmologist)* 119, 130
Watts, Mr. F. *(Senior Chief MLSO)* 149
Waugh, Nurse Janet 67
Webb, Laura *(Needle Mistress)* 38, 39
Webbs of Exning *(Contractor)* 45, 74
Wedgewood, Sister (Ward Sister) 110, 129, 149
Wells 42, 46
Welply, Dr. M. *(House Surgeon)* 66, 71, 75, 87, 101, 131
West London Teaching Hospital, Hammersmith 66
West, Dr. Roger *(Consultant in Public Health Medicine)* 175, 180
West Suffolk County Council 9, 53, 62, 77, 83, 94, 101, 104, 130
West Suffolk Health Authority 4, 145, 146, 149-151, 154, 156, 163, 164, 166, 171, 173, 175, 178-185
West Suffolk Hospital 105, 125, 131, 135, 143, 146, 165, 173, 175, 179, 182-185
West Suffolk HMC 10, 117
Wheeler, Mr. Jimmy *(Board of Guardians/House Committee member)* 37, 67, 73
White, Mr. *(Public Assistance Officer)* 53
White, Sister *(Ward Sister)* 111
White, Dr. Todd *(RHB Medical Department)* 83
White, Dr. Bobby Hall *(Medical Staff)* 66
Whitehouse, Dr. *(Consultant Pathologist)* 93
White Lodge EMS Hospital 9, 59-82
Whitwell, Mr. Stephen *(Health Authority member)* 179
Wiggin, Mr. J. O. *(Relieving Officer)* 53
Wilkinson, Dr. I. M. W. *(Consultant Neurologist)* 152
Wilkinson, Mrs. Kate *(District Nursing Advisor)* 163, 180
Williams, Dr. I. P *(Consultant Radiologist)* 93, 126, 139
Williams, Mrs. Lesley *(Senior Nurse Tutor)* 160
Williamson, Mr. R. *(Consultant ENT Surgeon)* 72, 75, 88, 93, 102
Wilson, Miss Diana *(Trainee Cook)* 114
Wings for Victory 71
Wiseman, Mr. A. D. *(Cook)* 39
Withers, Mr.J. R. *(Poet)* 32-33
Witley, Mr. B. M. *(Group Fire Officer)* 97, 130
Woodlands Hospital, Norfolk 67

Woodnough, Miss E. J. *(Ward Sister)* 159
Woods, Dr. G. *(Consultant Radiologist)* 152
Workhouse 13, 14, 21, 22, 25-34, 35, 37-40, 42-48, 49, 53-55, 66, 115, 132, 145, 167-170
Workhouse Master 30, 38 (see also Masters)
Work Study 101, 103, 105, 107-109, 112, 113, 129, 130, 135
"Working for Patients" - see NHS & Community Care Act 1990
Wright, Mr. H. *(Porter)* 57
W. R. V. S. 61, 96, 158

X-Ray Department 61, 62, 66, 68, 75, 76, 89, 93, 95, 100, 138, 139, 143, 144

York 8
Youngs, Mr. A. W. *(Group Secretary)* 87, 115

Zimmern, Dr. Ron *(Consultant in Public Health Medicine)* 175